Alchemy Amino Acids

The Power of Amino Acids in Mood and Health

Vanita Dahia

First published by Vanita Dahia 2019
Copyright © Vanita Dahia

ISBN
Print: 978-0-6481789-3-4
EBook: 978-0-6481789-2-7

Vanita Dahia is author of this work. The information in this book is based on the authors experience and opinions. Any references in this book have been noted and acknowledged. Any breaches will be rectified in further editions of this book. All rights reserved. Enquiries should be made through the publisher.

Cover design: Kev Howlett
Layout and typesetting: Busybird Publishing
Editor: Vanita Dahia

Busybird Publishing
2/118 Para Road
Montmorency, Victoria
Australia 3094

What do you call an acid with an attitude?

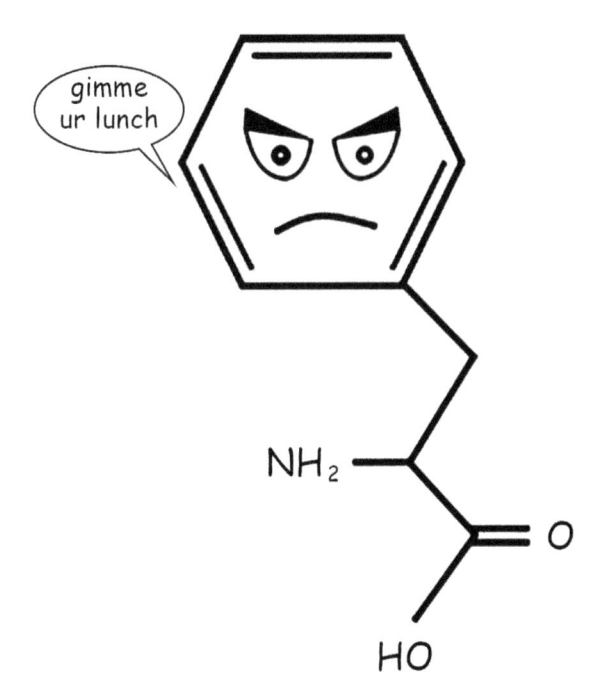

A-mean oh acid
Nerdy Humor by Sydney Grubb

Testimonials

HealthWise® amino acids are proud to be associated with the pioneer of compounding amino acids. Vanita Dahia, who is, without doubt, one of the most inspiring and well researched compounding pharmacist, practitioner and natural health advocate in Australia.

We are delighted to be able to contribute to Vanita's newest publication and look forward to being part of her future research projects.
   Carmel Krpan – Director Krpan Industries
   Ilve Hunt- Adv Dip HSC,
   DRM, researcher Amino Acid Compendium

There is an increasing incidence of epidemic proportions of calorie rich, nutrient poor diets contributing to many illnesses in the millennial to the post war generations, ranging from metabolic syndromes to nutrigenomics related diseases. Vanita Dahia's book will be an essential compendium to the experienced and the novice practitioner of integrative medicine. I am grateful she has contributed her vast knowledge of amino acid in a practical and digestible format.
   Dr Nathan Francis, Integrative Medical Doctor, Perth

After her first book, Alchemy of the Mind, Vanita has done it again with Alchemy of Amino Acids. This book just like the first one contains all the information one would ever need to know if they were interested in a complete analysis of the functions of amino acids, how to determine their balance in the body, how to adjust them if out of balance, thus affecting permanent resolution of symptoms in a natural way.

I highly recommend this book to all practitioners as a worthy addition to their arsenal.

John Catsicas – Compounding Pharmacist, Melbourne, Australia

Gratitude for Vanita Dahia's ongoing contribution to educating us all, professionals and public alike.

Vanita's vast knowledge, wisdom and many years experience as a Compounding Chemist, Naturopath, Practitioner and Consultant uniquely qualifies her as an expert.

Through her latest eBook Alchemy of Amino Acids, Vanita has once again demonstrated why she serves as advisor to doctors and laboratories. I call her the doctors' doctor.

Dr Ari Diskin, Chiropractic Doctor, Melbourne

Excellent companion for all Integrative Medicine practitioners.

Next to vitamins and minerals, amino acids are essential building blocks that play a huge part in clinical medicine.

Vanita Dahia has done it again with this long-awaited book Alchemy of Amino Acids, an essential guide to the use of amino acids in the functional approach to physical and mental disorders. This book gives step by step guidance to each amino acid explaining the physiological function, deficiency syndromes and how to use them therapeutically in clinical practice. Huge gratitude and appreciation.

Dr Margaret Jiin Ngu MBBS, FACNEM, FAMAC, MSE(Psych)

Vanita, I admire your passion and commitment in assisting health practitioners world-wide in understanding the power of amino acids for health conditions.

Congratulations on yet another book, Alchemy of Amino Acids. This book has helped me finally understand amino acids as it is it so easy to understand, implement the essential information and stay current. I mandate that everyone has a copy of this book, a great training tool.

Mary Cavvagion, Director Nutripath Pathology Services, Melbourne, Australia

Contents

Objective of Alchemy of Amino Acids	1
Introduction to Amino Acids	3
Value of Amino Acids	11
Amino Acid Utilization	15
Classification of Amino Acids	19
Materia Medica of Amino Acids	29
Benefits, clinical use, dosage ...	29
Alanine	30
Beta Alanine	31
Arginine	32
Arginine alpha-ketoglutarate (AAKG)	35
Asparagine	35
Aspartic acid	37
D-Aspartic acid (D-AA)	38
Carnitine	39
Acetyl – l-carnitine	41
Choline	42
Citrulline	44
Creatine	45
Cysteine	46
N-acetyl-Cysteine	48
N-acetyl D glucosamine (NAG)	50
L-Glucosamine HCl	52

GABA	54
Glutamine	57
Glycine	59
Inositol	61
Histidine	62
Isoleucine	64
Leucine	65
Lysine	67
Methionine	68
Ornithine	70
Phenylalanine	71
Proline	73
Serine	75
Taurine	76
L-Theanine	78
Threonine	79
Tryptophan	81
Tyrosine	83
Valine	86
Therapeutic Value of Amino Acids	89
Testing of Amino Acids	107
Interpretation of Amino Acid Analysis	115
Treatment – Balancing Amino Acid levels	155
Acknowledgments	181
References	183

Objective of Alchemy of Amino Acids

Health practitioners are bombarded with technical and research data on Amino Acids. The objective of Alchemy of Amino Acids is to provide easy to read charts detailing what it means to have low or high level of an amino acid, how to read a lab report, what it means clinically and how to custom compound a prescription based on a lab report.

In the past, some health professionals and amino acid suppliers have formulated prescriptive protocols for the patient loosely based on their specific algorithms.

I have for the last 30 years worked at developing an easy to implement compounding algorithm that is practical, clinically relevant with positive therapeutic outcomes My specific template for compounding is by no means conclusive but has worked for me over the years. I saw amazing positive therapeutic outcomes from my compounded amino acid formulae. I will show you how to tweak a formula to suit your patient's needs. I feel obliged to share what has worked for me and am open to opinions and suggestions to enhance the health of the patient.

Introduction to Amino Acids

"People crave laughter as if it were an essential amino acid."
Patch Adams

What's the big deal about Amino Acids?

Amino acids are essential to life. Without amino acids, we will have no genes. After all, the sequence of amino acids maps out our ancestral hereditary, makes every cell in the body grow as it is our DNA and RNA. Amino acids are needed for practically every biochemical pathway within the body.

Next to minerals, amino acids are essential to life. The common denominator to cellular health are two very important categories of nutrients – trace elements also known as tissue salts and amino acids. These are essential to life! The foundation nutrients need to be in place before addition of vitamins, trace elements, herbs or pharmaceutical drug.

I am passionate about balancing body chemistries and in particular amino acids because I have seen the immediate therapeutic benefit of taking a single amino acid.

> *"The basic structure of proteins is quite simple: they are formed by hooking together in a chain discrete subunit called amino acids"*
> Michael Behe.

Amino acids are essential to life.

Amino acids are central to virtually every function of the human body. The pool of amino acids is highly dynamic, changing moment by moment by shifting the flow of metabolic pathways in response to multiple physiological signals.

The word "protein" is derived from the Greek "protos," meaning "first," a designating its prominence in life.

Scientific research has demonstrated that conditions as varied as chemical sensitivities, cardiovascular disease, macular degeneration, bone disorders and insomnia are associated with amino acid imbalances. [1] The raft of health conditions associated with amino acid metabolism is a result of the countless physiological processes that these molecules are involved in. The production of neurotransmitters, hormones, nitric oxide, urea, antioxidants, connective tissue and ATP are just a few examples. They are essential and important in neurotransmitter function, pH regulation, cholesterol metabolism, pain control, detoxification, and control of inflammation.

What do carnivores, vegetarians and omnivores all have in common? They all require protein in order to sustain and optimize life. Protein is the second most abundant substance in our bodies after water. It constitutes ¾ of the dry weight of most body cells. It is involved in the biochemical structure of genes, blood, tissue, muscle, collagen, skin, hair, and nails, and is a major constituent of all the many hormones, enzymes, nutrient carriers, infection-fighting antibodies, neurotransmitters and other chemical messengers in the body. This continuous process of building and regeneration is necessary for life and requires a non-stop supply of protein.[2]

In free form or linked as peptides they are components of growth hormones, DNA and RNA genetics and assume important roles in practically every metabolic pathway in the body, manufacture of hormones and work synergistically with specific vitamins, minerals and trace elements in maintenance of physiology.

Amino acids comprise the building blocks of the proteins found in structural tissues of the body. Amino acids are in a constant flux due to total body protein dynamics. They are 20 peptide forming essential and non-essential amino acids required for enzyme, structural and transporter proteins. Amino acids are required to load RNA and DNA for protein synthesis.

Catabolism of amino acids increases to support gluconeogenesis (breakdown of muscle tissue) for energy sources. Insulin down regulates gene expression of amino acid catabolism. Glucocorticoids on the other hand, up regulate amino acid catabolism.

When amino acids are catabolized during exercise, ammonia that is formed must be removed. There are 40,000 different proteins found in the body and they are all made from 20 amino acids required by the body for the production of proteins such as:

- Muscle
- Collagen
- Hormones
- Enzymes
- Neurotransmitters

The knowledge of amino acids is most helpful in the field of medicine because of its constant need for food during health as well as illness.

Amino Acids possess both physiological and pharmacological actions. Amino acids are needed to produce transport proteins such as albumin, transferrin and sex hormone binding globulin.

Amino acids do not function on their own. Each biochemical process in the body is a complex inter-relationship between amino acids and with other nutrients which act as co-factors.

Ancestry, DNA, Genetics and Amino Acids

We know that dog give birth to little pups and sharks to little sharks and not another creature. **Why is this so?** The answer lies in a molecule called deoxyribonucleic acid (DNA), which contains the biological instructions that make each species unique. DNA, along with the instructions it contains, is passed from adult organisms to their offspring during reproduction.

DNA, our genetic signature is found in organisms called eukaryotes. DNA is found inside the nucleus of each cell. Organisms have many DNA molecules per cell, each DNA molecule must be tightly packaged. This packaged form of the DNA is called a chromosome.

During DNA replication, DNA unwinds so it can be copied. At other times in the cell cycle, DNA also unwinds so that its instructions can be used to make proteins and for other biological processes. But during cell division, DNA is in its compact chromosome form to enable transfer to new cells.

DNA and RNA, the genes are made up 4 primary amino acid sequences. To form a strand of DNA, nucleotides are linked into chains, with the phosphate and sugar groups alternating. The four bases found in DNA are Adenine (A), Cytosine (C), Guanine (G) And Thymine (T). These four bases are attached to the sugar-phosphate to form the complete nucleotide. Adenine pairs with thymine and guanine pairs with cytosine.

Proteins are built from a basic set of 20 amino acids, but there are only four bases. Simple calculations show that a minimum of three bases is required to encode at least 20 amino acids. Genetic experiments showed that an amino acid is in fact encoded by a group of three bases, or codon. The code is non-overlapping.

Types of DNA: There are three main types of DNA tests that are available: Y-chromosome (Y-DNA) tests for the direct paternal line, mitochondrial DNA (mtDNA) tests for the direct maternal line, and autosomal DNA (atDNA) tests for finding matches on all your ancestral lines.

Expression of genes: Transcription is the first step of gene expression, in which a particular segent of DNA is copied into RNA (especially mRNA) by the enzyme RNA polymerase. Both DNA and RNA are nucleic acids, which use base pairs of nucleotides as a complementary language. If the cell has a nucleus, the RNA may be further processed.

Growth Hormone and Amino Acids

Growth Hormone is a stress hormone that raises the concentration of glucose and free fatty acids. It also stimulates production of IGF-1.

Growth hormone injections are synthesized of 191 single-chain polypeptide amino acids, stored and secreted by somatotropic cells within the anterior pituitary gland. Specific amino acids, such as Arginine, Lysine and Ornithine, can stimulate growth hormone (GH) release when infused intravenously or administered orally.

Oral supplementation of Lysine and Ornithine, can stimulate growth hormone promoting greater gains in muscle mass and strength.[3]

Peptides - Innovations in Amino Acid Therapy

The use of peptide injections has been popularized in the body building industry. Abuse and subsequent bad press of peptide use makes it a prescription injection item and therefore well-regulated.

Amino acids are building blocks of protein which essentially acts as a scaffolding that mitigates all cell reactions in the body. DNA makes RNA which is composed of peptides and proteins. Peptides therefore of the building blocks and proteins are signaling molecules. Is an arbitrary measure a chain of 50 amino acids or less are considered peptides whereas 50 amino acids and more make up proteins?

Peptides are short chains of amino acid monomers linked by peptide (amide) bonds. The covalent chemical bonds are formed when the carboxyl group of one amino acid reacts with the amino group of another. Peptide hormones refer to any hormone derived from amino acids.

When peptides form a long chain of amino acids, they become proteins. When they are in a short chain of amino acids, they are able to penetrate the top layer of our skin and send signals to our cells to let them know how to function. One important protein in our skin is collagen.

Peptide supplementation is fast becoming a solution to a variety of health, fitness, and age-related concerns. Peptides have been around long before the recent media brought it to our attention through use in elite sport. The simple science of amino acids linked together, via peptide bonds, bring to life this now common word—peptides.

The conditions in which peptides recommended and well published art in cancer, metabolic disorders and inflammatory conditions. The use of peptides has now been expanded in the mould, Lyme and chronic inflammatory diseases. The study of peptides has been reported in the 1990s to stimulate growth hormone secretion from the pituitary. In 1995, peptides GHRP6, a gruelin hormone has also been shown to stimulate growth hormone release.[4]

The benefits of peptides in health and well-being include:

- Weight – fat tissue reduction, weight management
- Skin – peptides in topical applications has been shown to increase skin elasticity, texture and tightness, hair texture
- Muscle tone – increase lean muscle mass, strength
- Energy – increase ATP production and emotional stability
- Bone density – improves bone strength
- Libido – increase sexual potency and frequency
- Cardiovascular health – improve cardiovascular strength and blood pressure, kidney function cholesterol
- Immunity – improve healing

What do Depression, Sleep, Heart Disease, and Detoxification Imbalances have in Common?

Many cell functions can be restored by providing amino acids to assist neurotransmitter hormone synthesis. Hepatic and gastrointestinal detoxification reactions are improved when amino acids required for conjugation are available. Sulphur amino acids are needed to supply adequate glutathione.

The common denominator is its association with amino acid levels.

- Low Tyrosine or Phenylalanine can result in abnormal levels of mood-regulating dopamine and catecholamines.
- Low Ornithine, Glycine and Serine may impair sleep onset and duration. Thought its only Tryptophan and GABA supporting sleep?
- Both low Taurine and high Homocysteine have been associated with cardiovascular problems.
- Low levels of Methionine, Glycine, and Glutathione are implicated in liver detoxification and clearance of toxic substances from the body.

Value of Amino Acids

Amino acids are absolutely valuable in practically every physiological function in the body. It is possible to ease pain, soothe anxiety, and improve memory simply by taking amino acids.

The benefits of taking amino-acids to improve your health can hardly be overstated. All the body tissues - every muscle, hair, nail, enzyme, and brain cell is made from amino-acids. They are central to the bio-chemistry of your body.

Amino Acids play a major role in nearly every chemical process that affects both physical and mental function. As a result, amino acids have more diverse functions than any other nutrient group, including:

- Cellular energy production
- Formation of ligaments, tendons, and bones
- Formation of antibodies
- Formation and regulation of enzymes and blood transport proteins

Amino acids play central roles both as building blocks of proteins and as intermediates in metabolism. They not only catalyze all (or most) of the reactions in living cells, they control virtually all cellular processes.

Deficiencies and excesses of these vital molecules therefore lead to physiological impairment which is exhibited in a wide variety of clinical symptoms.

Amino acids are required in many physiological functions:
- Gastrointestinal
- Detoxification
- Cardiovascular
- musculoskeletal
- Neurological
- Endocrine
- Oxidative stress
- Nutrient Adequacy

Symptoms and Conditions associated with Amino Acid Imbalances

- Allergies
- Anxiety & panic attacks
- Arthritis
- Bile insufficiency
- Cardiovascular disease
- Chemical exposure and sensitivities
- Connective tissue and bone disorders
- Depression
- Diabetes or insulin dysregulation
- Eating disorders
- Estrogen imbalances (low methylated estrogens); increased cancer risk
- Fatigue
- Hypertension
- Hypoglycaemia
- Inflammatory conditions
- Insomnia
- Low libido
- Macular degeneration
- Neurological conditions (e.g. autism, dementia, histapenia, schizophrenia)

Value of Amino Acids

- Migraines
- Muscle atrophy & weakness
- Negative nitrogen balance
- Poor wound healing
- Thyroid conditions
- Viral infections (e.g. cold sores, shingles)

Amino Acid Utilization

Amino acid utilization is tissue and time-dependent. During sleep, amino acids from the blood stream are used for tissue repair, detoxification and restoration. Amino acids are broken down from skeletal muscle and oxidized for energy in the morning upon awakening.

During the allergy season, gastric mucosal cells have a large demand for histamine to supply the precursor formation of histamine, a neurotransmitter.

During times of stress, the demand for Tryptophan by serotonergic cells in the intestine and brain is increased.

High plasma essential amino acid levels show you the increased release due to catabolism or decreased utilization.

High intestinal transit rates can also decrease protein digestions deficiency.

Exercise in injury have a higher need for carbohydrates; the intake of 100 g of carbohydrates one hour after resistance exercise has been shown to decrease the release of amino acids in the blood.[5]

Arginine has been shown to act similar to and in some cases replace Sildenafil (Viagra) for restoring erectile function and a sagging libido. It has also been found to increase sperm count.

Breakdown products of bone in Hydroxyproline may prove more advantageous for assessing bone loss than the standard bone density test.

Boosting energy levels in the brain with Phenylalanine and Tyrosine is key to weight loss.

Melatonin and Tryptophan have established themselves as multipurpose nutrients to improve sleep, defuse anxiety and slow down the aging process. Recent studies show promise for the use of Tryptophan in the treatment of autism.

Homocysteine has gained recognition as a major independent risk indicator for cardiovascular disease. New research suggests it may also pretend neural tube defects, sickle cell disease, rectal polyps, and liver failure, and may contribute to depression, dementia and loss of brain function in the elderly.

Tyrosine can help cocaine and alcohol abusers kick their habits and combat the effects of stress, narcolepsy, chronic fatigue, and ADD.

Amino acid blood levels are increasingly serving as important indicators of physical and mental illnesses. They provide major nutritional and biochemical clues for more effective treatment.

Carnitine has been shown to offer significant protection against the common side effects of Depakote (a popular drug used for seizures and psychotic disorders). Its derivative N-acetyl-carnitine may surpass the metabolic potency of carnation in the brain, where it has been found to slow the progression of Alzheimer's disease.

Scientific evidence continues to mount showing N-acetyl Cysteine to be perhaps the most powerful detoxifier in the body. It is now found in every emergency room as an antidote to overdose cases and as well can render harmless everyday environmental toxins.

New, modified GABA compounds such as gabapentin (Neurontin) and tigabine (Gabitril) are producing improved uptake in the brain and appear to be important products in the control of seizures and anxiety disorders. Early studies indicate GABA may also be correlated to a decrease in benign prostatic hypertrophy.

Research with Serine compounds show that blocking Serine metabolism may serve to prevent autoimmune activity present in psychoses.[6]

Glutamic and Aspartic acids create additional neurotoxic damage in the brain following stroke. New drug that block the action of the excretory amino acid transporters (EAATs) have recently been approved.[7]

BCAAs promote optimal muscle growth and improve performance; additionally they also offer promise for staving off muscle loss as we age.

Classification of Amino Acids

Classifying amino acids based on structure, acidity, mineral content, function, or availability in the diet is necessary to establish the nature and properties of each amino acid and how it might work synergistically with other amino acids as a therapeutic tool.

Just as we compartmentalize our jobs or location of residence or financial status against others to establish a value system or system of importance, amino acids too would be best compartmentalized to develop a further understanding of these vital nutrients in health.

All amino acids have a central carbon atom surrounded by a hydrogen atom, a carboxyl group (COOH), an amino group (NH2), and an R-group. It is the R-group or side chain that differs between the 20 amino acids.

Chemically speaking, an amino acid is a carboxylic acid which has an amine group attached to it. All amino acids found in proteins have this basic structure, differing only in the structure of the R-group or the side chain.

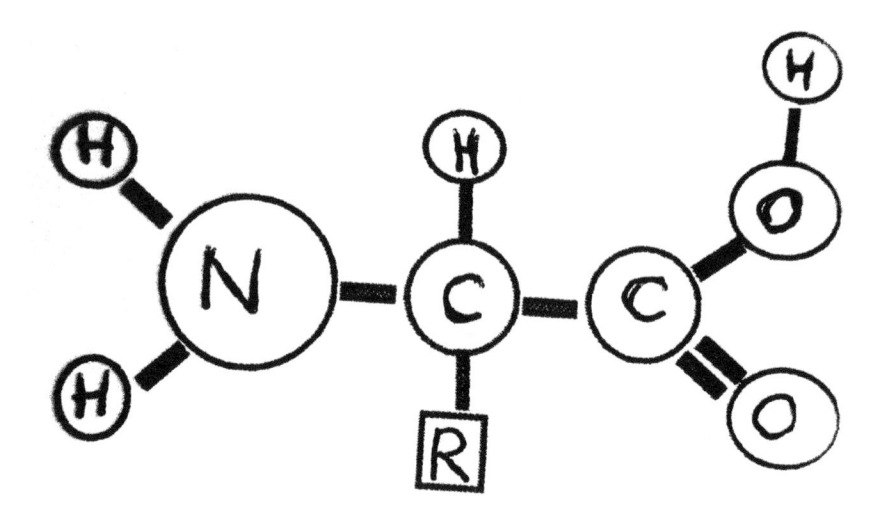

In proteins, only the L-isomer is found in nature.

Classification of amino acids are necessary to identify its actions, where is synthesized or derived from or its physiological characteristics.

Amino Acids can be classified into categories based on:
- Essential value i.e. found in the diet and needs to be synthesised
- Conditionally essential
- Nonessential
- Basic
- Function i.e. glucogenic or ketogenic
- Isomers i.e. stereoisomers of D and L-forms
- Hydrophobicity
- Size
- Charge
- Alcoholicity
- Aromaticity
- Different combinations of small/large, charged/uncharged, polar/nonpolar properties

Isomers

Every amino acid molecule contains at least one amino group (-NH2) and carboxyl group (-COOH). Amino acids are in either an "L" or "D" configuration. The difference of isomers is determined by which side of the molecule the amino group (-NH2) is attached.

Amino Acids exist on earth to stereoisomers namely L and D forms. L amino acids are utilized in human metabolism. Most amino acids are supplemented as L-forms.

Specific isomers may be of value for different therapeutic functions. L-Phenylalanine, for example, is an active precursor of Dopamine and PEA whereas DL-forms of Phenylalanine has been shown to be effective as an analgesic.

Basic Amino Acids have basic side chains at neutral pH. These are Arginine (Arg), Lysine (Lys), and Histidine (His). Their side chains contain nitrogen and resemble ammonia, which is a base.

Essential amino acids must be derived from the diet. Amino acids formed in other metabolic pathways are sometimes dispensable and called non-essential amino acids.

Limitations on the rates of amino acids that are technically **non-essential** become essential to maintain optimal wellness under specific diseases or conditions are called **conditionally essential** amino acids.

Amino acids may belong to more than one category of classification. For example, amino acids may be classified into:

Hydrophobic

Aliphatic	Alanine, Leucine, Isoleucine, Valine
Aromatic	Phenylalanine, Tyrosine, Tryptophan, (Histadine)

Hydrophilic

Polar	Aspartic Acid, Glycine
Alcoholic	Serine, Threonine, (Tyrosine)
Charged	Arginine, Lysine, Aspartic Acid, Glutamine, (Histadine)

Inbetween:

Sulphur-containing	Methionine, Cysteine
Special	Glycine, Proline (cyclic)

Some amino acids are formed by reaction by the addition of chemical groups such as hydroxyl-Proline and hydroxyl-Lysine needed for the production of collagen.

More specifically, amino acid classes are as follows:

Essential amino acids

- Histamine
- Isoleucine
- Leucine
- Lysine
- Methionine
- Phenylalanine
- Threonine
- Tryptophan
- Valine

Conditionally essential amino acids

- Arginine
- Glutamine
- Glycine
- Taurine
- Non-essential amino acids
- Alanine
- Asparagine
- Aspartic acid
- Cysteine
- Glutamic acid
- Proline

Amino acid derivatives

Some amino acids may be hydroxylated such as Lysine and Proline after they are incorporated into polypeptide or protein structure. Lysine becomes Hydroxylysine.

Other examples of amino acid derivatives:

- Alpha amino butyric acid
- Hydroxyproline
- Methyl-histidine
- Ornithine
- Citrulline

Therapeutic Classification of Amino Acids

Glucogenic Amino Acids form metabolic intermediates which form Glucose after they have lost their amino group (usually by transamination). Glucogenic Amino Acids facilitate the body's production of Energy (after they have been metabolized to Glucose within the liver). Glucogenic Amino Acids are metabolized to Glucose within the Liver - this conversion is catalyzed by Glucagon (hormone).

- Aspartate
- Asparagine
- Arginine
- Phenylalanine
- Tyrosine
- Isoleucine
- Methionine
- Valine
- Glutamine
- Glutamate
- Proline
- Histidine
- Alanine
- Serine
- Cysteine
- Glycine
- Threonine
- Tryptophan

Ketogenic Amino Acids are Amino Acids that form Ketones after losing their amino group.

- Isoleucine
- Leucine
- Threonine
- Tryptophan
- Lysine
- Phenylalanine

- Tyrosine
- Sulphur-based Amino Acids include Sulphur in their chemical structure which includes:
- Cysteine
- Cystine
- Methionine
- Taurine

Certain classes of amino acids have their unique physiological function which affects metabolic load.

Large neutral amino acids- Tryptophan, Tyrosine, Phenylalanine, Leucine, Isoleucine, Methionine can compete for intestinal absorption and transport at the blood brain barrier.

Basic amino acids – histamine Lysine, Arginine are abundant in histones and tend bind to negatively charged DNA. Imbalances in these amino acids have the potential to affect methylation processes or present as DNA polymorphisms.

Branched Chain Amino Acids (BCAAs)

Branched chain amino acids are essential to life and are metabolized by muscle tissue.

They are predominantly Valine, Isoleucine and Leucine.

Valine deficiency is associated with neurological defects.

Valine RDA 24mg/kg/day i.e. 1680mg in 70kg adult

Isoleucine deficiency is associated with muscle tremors.

Recommended dose of Isoleucine is RDA 19mg/kg/day i.e.1330mg in 70kg adult

Leucine RDA 42mg/kg/day e.g. 2 940mg in 70kg adult

Isoleucine & Valine are glucogenic whereas Leucine is ketogenic.

BCAAs are commonly used in endurance training where the requirement is increased due to oxidation of BCAAs. There is, however, a fair amount of speculation around increased protein requirements for exercise.[8]

BCAA's are the most easily oxidized type of amino acid in the skeletal muscles and serves as an important energy substrate when carbohydrate becomes exhausted after a prolonged exercise, as the contribution rate of fat as an energy source increases.

Intake of BCAA's can lower the concentration of serotonin, a central fatigue substance, during endurance exercise, which subsequently can reduce the concentrations of muscle damage substances such as Creatinine kinase (CK) and Lactate dehydrogenase (LDH), muscle damage substances and enhance exercise performance; the higher the ammonia concentration, the higher the LDH concentration is. In addition, a less secretion of FFA leads to a reduced secretion of LDH.

Glucose is used as a major energy source during exercise but is replaced with FFA in more than one hour of endurance exercise. Therefore, the intake of the BCAA is presumed to help contribute to enhancing exercise performance by exerting its influence on fatigue substances, muscle damage substances, and energy metabolism substances. It is therefore recommended to supplement with BCAA's during athletic training and body building.

A depletion of BCAA's are associated with mental retardation, ataxia, hypoglycemia, spinal muscle atrophy, rash, vomiting, excess movements, tardive dyslexia, amyotrophic lateral sclerosis, and other muscular degenerative disorders.

A greater need to supplementation with BCAA's is recommended in times of stress, surgery, trauma, cirrhosis, infections, fever & starvation.

BCAA supplementation has the potential to reduce the need for steroid use.

Person Centric Variation of Amino Acids

Factors like poor digestion function, improper use of medications such as antacids or acid blockers, increased stress responses, poor eating habits, and aging can affect the body's ability to provide essential nutrients at a tissue level. As a result, adequate protein intake does not ensure an optimal amino acid supply for physiological purposes.

Metabolic disorders may interfere with amino acid utilization, such as genetic polymorphisms, nutrient deficiencies or toxicant abnormalities.

Amino acids status may vary between different individuals due to:

- Age – levels may decline with age. Lysine and Tryptophan concentrations may change approximately 30% from birth to adolescence
- Auto-immune diseases, infection increases immune system demand for amino acids
- Inherited metabolic diseases - phenylketonuria, maple syrup urine disease, homocysteinuria, tyrosinemia, hyperphenylalaninemia
- Defects of biopterin cofactor regeneration
- Dietary protein intake
- Amino acid needs vary in respect of nitrogen balance
- Digestion - Protein digestion affects amino acid absorption. Hypochlohydria may impair digestion of protein and subsequently deplete amino acid levels to tissues
- Excessive exercise
- Injury
- Protein supplements used by strength building routines
- Amino acid transport - levels of amino acids are influenced by transporters
- High intestinal transit rates can decrease protein digestion
- Genetic polymorphisms
- Toxicant abnormalities
- Nutrient deficiencies

Person centric variation of amino acid status and nutrient need requires a personalized treatment approach or compounded amino acids.

Materia Medica of Amino Acids

Benefits, clinical use, dosage, side effects, contraindications of each Amino Acid

The term materia medica reminds me of learning to understand raw materials within the science of pharmacognosy during my pharmacy training years. The science of pharmacognosy is obsolete, however essential, really get an understanding of each raw material used in medications. I remember in an exam, being blindfolded and tasting a finger that had been dipped in a raw material powder to identify the components such as terpinoids, alkaloids, acidity, and so on. It is based on these properties that the characteristics, therapeutic function, side effects, dosage, adverse reactions, contraindications, can be determined. Materia Medica, therefore is the science of each raw material, and in this context, the science of amino acids!

Each individual amino acid has its own therapeutic benefit, optimal dosage, side effects, adverse effects and therapeutic usage. Amino acids appear in our diet as a synergistic blend, perhaps some amino acids more dominant than others. Glutamine for example is the most abundant amino acid found in most protein sources. Therapeutically, individual amino acids may be used for specific conditions such as Lysine for cold sores or Arginine or cardiovascular health.

Alanine

Also known as: L-alpha-Alanine; (S)-Alanine; L-2-Aminopropionic acid; (S)-2-Aminopropionic acid; L-α-Aminopropionic acid

Primary use: sugar and acid metabolism

Alanine is a proteinogenic primary amino acid while beta-Alanine is a non-proteinogenic amino acid. Alanine is a **non-essential amino acid** used in protein synthesis and the regeneration of glucose within the liver via the glucose–Alanine cycle. This amino acid is synthesized by reductive amination of pyruvate, and participates in sugar and acid metabolism.

Fatigue

Alanine helps your body **convert the simple sugar called glucose into energy** you need, while eliminating excess toxins from the liver.[9]

Immunity

Alanine increases immunity and providing energy for brain and central nervous system, let alone the muscle tissue. Alanine plays a central role in glucose-Alanine cycle taking place between tissues and liver.

Benign prostatic hyperplasia

Prostate gland fluid contains this amino acid, hence Alanine may help treat benign prostatic hyperplasia, enlargement of the prostate gland.

Cholesterol management

Alanine in combination with Arginine and Glycine have been shown to have a cholesterol-reducing effect.

It can be obtained from various sources like seafood, meat, dairy products, caseinate, fish, egg, lactalbumin and gelatin (for animal sources) and nuts, beans, whey, soy, brown rice, brewer's yeast, corn, bran, whole grains and legumes (for vegetable sources). Among these sources, Alanine is highly concentrated in meat products.

Beta Alanine

Also known as: b-Alanine, β-Alanine, carnosine precursor

Primary Use: muscle Gain and Exercise

This is the only naturally occurring β-amino acid in the brain. It is a **component of carnosine, Anserine and of pantothenic acid (vitamin B5)** which is itself a component of coenzyme A. These three are called dipeptides which contain the beta-Alanine. They are richly stored in meats like fish, pork, beef and chicken.

When beta-Alanine is ingested, it turns into the molecule carnosine, which acts as an acid buffer in the body. Carnosine is stored in cells and released in response to drops in pH. Increased stores of carnosine can protect against diet-induced drops in pH (which might occur from ketone production in ketosis), as well as offer protection from exercise-induced lactic acid production.

Carnosine appears to be an **antioxidant and anti-aging** compound. This means that increasing the amount of beta-Alanine will increase the total carnosine concentration in the muscles.[10]

Beta-Alanine is metabolized to acetic acid, and in plants and micro-organisms it is formed from Aspartic acid. Beta-Alanine can aid lean-mass gain. Carnosine appears to be an antioxidant and anti-aging compound. Beta-Alanine is a modified version of the amino acid Alanine.

Fatigue

Increasing carnosine will help reduce fatigue among athletes and elevate overall muscular strength. Beta-Alanine can also improve both anaerobic and aerobic endurances.

Enhance muscular endurance

Beta-Alanine has been shown to improve moderate- to high-intensity cardiovascular exercise performance.

Dosage

Standard daily dose: 2–5 g. While beta-Alanine is a popular ingredient in pre-workout formulae, supplementation is actually not timing-dependent.

Large doses of beta-Alanine may cause a tingling feeling called paresthesia, a neuropathic sensation of pain most especially if it exceeds 10 mg per kilo of body weight, although this varies per individual.

Arginine

Also known as: L-Arginine

Primary Usage: muscle Gain and exercise

Other uses: cardiovascular

Arginine HCl is a synthetically manufactured form of Arginine that combines the amino acid with a hydrogen chloride molecule. Hydrogen chloride is combined with Arginine to make the supplement more palatable and to enhance its absorption by the digestive system.

Arginine HCL and Athletic Performance

One of the main effects of Arginine is that it causes vasodilation, by stimulating the smooth muscle endothelial cells that line the blood vessels to produce a compound called nitric oxide.

Nitric oxide stimulates blood vessels to relax and expand, increasing the flow of blood and oxygen to the muscles during bouts of intense exercise, especially resistance training.

An increase in blood flow and oxygen delivery during exercise may enhance performance, allowing muscles to produce more strength and delaying the onset of exercise induced fatigue.

Arginine HCL and Hormone Production

Arginine is an important catalyst for the production of human growth hormone, or HGH.

When ingested, Arginine HCl stimulates the anterior pituitary gland to release HGH, increasing plasma levels of HGH circulating throughout the body.

Naturally elevated levels of HGH have many benefits, including an increase in muscle recovery and repair, regulation of metabolism, body fat reduction, and the optimal functioning of the heart and kidneys.

Taking Arginine in conjunction with other amino acids like Ornithine, may enhance this effect. Studies suggest **2 Arginine:1 Ornithine to stimulate HGH production**

Arginine HCL may have a wide range of potential benefits beyond its use as a performance enhancer for athletes.[11]

MedlinePlus reports that possible benefits of Arginine HCL supplementation include improving surgery recovery time, treating congestive heart failure, reducing chest pain in coronary artery disease, reducing bladder inflammation, treating erectile dysfunction, improving kidney function, and maintaining a healthy body weight in individuals suffering from muscle-wasting diseases such as HIV.

Blood Flow

May increase blood flow secondary to activating nitric oxide. Implicated in reducing blood pressure.[12]

Side Effects

Arginine HCL may have adverse effects on individuals who have liver and kidney disease, as well as on some individuals recovering from a heart attack.

Arginine HCL may also upset the balance of potassium in the bloodstream.

With a potassium deficiency, Arginine may cause dehydration, nausea, stomach cramps and diarrhea. Monitor use with blood thinning medications.

Individuals with chronically low blood pressure are advised not to take Arginine, as it may lower blood pressure even further, leading to fatigue and dizziness.

Dosage

The recommended dosage of Arginine varies depending on the treatment.

The standard pre-workout dose for L-Arginine is 3-6g. To maintain elevated Arginine levels throughout the day, Arginine can be taken up to three times a day, with a combined dose total of 15-18g.

Note: L-Citrulline supplementation is more effective at maintaining elevated Arginine levels for long periods of time. Taking more than 10g of Arginine at once can result in gastrointestinal distress and diarrhea.

For congestive heart failure, MedlinePlus recommends doses ranging from 6g to 20g per day, which varies on a case-by-case basis.

For relieving chest pain caused by clogged arteries, 9 g to 28 g of Arginine is taken in equal increments three or four times daily.

Men suffering from erectile dysfunction may benefit from 5g of L-Arginine per day.

6 g per day is an effective dosage for improving physical performance.

Arginine alpha-ketoglutarate (AAKG)

AAKG is commonly found within pre-workout supplements as it has been shown to enhance performance. A study in the Journal of the International Society of Sports Nutrition suggested that AAKG may be able to significantly improve intra-workout performance by **supporting Creatine production**, **improving blood flow**, and **boosting nitric oxide levels** in the blood.

This suggests that AAKG may be able to help you extend your total fatigue time while boosting strength output.

Boost nitric oxide levels: AAKG is a nitric oxide booster, dilating vessels to increase intense pumps, better performance, and **greater muscle gain** and strength.

Build muscle mass: higher levels of nitric oxide may help to promote greater levels of muscle mass.[13]

AAKG has been suggested to be a potent **recovery aid,** promoting the healing of lean tissue.

Dosage: between 2,000 and 2,500 mg, based on physical activity level.

Asparagine

Also known as: (S)-2-Aminosuccinic acid 4-amide; alpha-Amino-succinamic acid; L-Aspartic acid 4-amide; (2S)-2-Amino-3-carbamoyl-propanoic acid

Primary Use: biosynthesis of glycoproteins

Asparagine is known worldwide as the first amino acid that was isolated from its natural source. Asparagine was isolated in 1806 from asparagus juice by Pierre Jean Robiquet and Louis-Nicolas Vauquelin.

Asparagine is a non-essential amino acid, a beta-amino derivative of Aspartic acid and plays an important role in the biosynthesis of glycoproteins and other proteins. A metabolic precursor to aspartate, Asparagine is a nontoxic carrier of residual ammonia to be eliminated from the body.

Asparagine is known for its key role in the **biosynthesis of glycoproteins**. In addition, it is also essential for the synthesis of many other proteins. Human nervous system also needs this amino acid to be able to maintain an equilibrium. Asparagine increases the resistance to fatigue and improves the smooth functioning of the liver. So, Asparagine benefits work best in the field of **nervine health and liver protection**.[14]

Currently, Asparagine is one of the twenty most common amino acids on our planet - one of the principal and the most abundant elements that help to transport nitrogen.

It can be produced in the liver and is recognized worldwide for its ability to help increase the resistance to **fatigue**, thus improving **athletic stamina**.

Neuronal development: involved in signaling, neuronal development and transmission across nerve ending.

This amino acid is actually an essential component of proteins involved in signaling, **neuronal development and transmission** across nerve ending. It is also necessary for transformation of amino acid from one form to another. In addition, Asparagine is known for its key role in the biosynthesis of glycoproteins, as well as in the synthesis of many other proteins.

People experiencing a deficiency of Asparagine may suffer from poor metabolism and show inability to manufacture and excrete urea, which is waste product of excess dietary protein. Such people thus may reveal symptoms like depression, confusion, and headaches. In addition, among the main benefits of Asparagine you can find the facts that it may help in metabolizing ammonia in the human body and enable proper functioning of the liver, as well as it enables a robust system resistant to fatigue.

Food sources of Asparagine

The most common typical dietary sources of this amino acid include beef, chicken, dairy products, seafood, and egg. As for vegetarians, they may find helpful to consume asparagus, soy, and whole grains to get more amino acid from them.

Aspartic acid

Also known as: L-Aspartic acid, D-Aspartic acid, L-aspartate

Primary Use: energy production

Aspartic Acid is a **non-essential amino acid** playing a major role in the energy cycle of your body. Besides, Aspartic acid also participates in the Ornithine cycle, in transamination reactions, as well as in the formation of pyrimidines, purines, carnosine, and Anserine.

This amino acid is necessary for **stamina, brain and neural health**. Aspartic acid is recognized as an important element removing excess toxins from the cells, especially ammonia that damages human liver, brain, and nervous system.

RNA and DNA

Important in the functioning of RNA and DNA, as well as in the production of immunoglobulin and antibody synthesis. It promotes transportation of minerals to the cells, which are essential to form healthy RNA and DNA, while strengthening the immune system through stimulating an increased production of immunoglobulins and antibodies.

Promote metabolism

Aspartate is believed to help your body promote a robust metabolism. This amino acid plays a key role in the citric acid cycle (also known as Krebs cycle), and has been used in depression and fatigue.

Chronic Fatigue Syndrome

Aspartic acid got its reputation for being a treatment substance for chronic fatigue and for the vital role it plays in generating cellular energy.

Cognition

It increases concentrations of NADH in the brain improving cognition. It is believed to boost up the production of chemicals necessary for proper mental functioning.

It is found in such food sources as dairy, beef, poultry, sugar cane and molasses. Individuals with diets low in protein or having eating disorders or malnutrition may suffer from the results of Aspartic acid deficiency like extreme fatigue or depression.

D-Aspartic acid (D-AA)

D-Aspartic acid is an amino acid regulator of testosterone synthesis and may act on a stimulatory receptor (NMDA). The benefits of D-AA are specific to it, and do not extend to Aspartic acid or L-aspartate.

Male fertility

D-AA shows promise in aiding male fertility by temporarily increasing testosterone. D-AA increases secretion of Gonadotropin releasing hormone (GnRH), Growth-Hormone releasing hormone (GHRH), and Prolactin Releasing Factors (PRFs) which cause releases of Luteinizing hormone (LH) and Follicle-Stimulating Hormone (FSH), Growth Hormone (GH), and Prolactin, respectively.

Pineal Hormones

D-Aspartate acts as a regulatory factor for melatonin secretion. L-Aspartate also has the ability to suppress melatonin synthesis.

Boost testosterone

There has been an induction (increase) in the enzyme that degrades D-Aspartic acid, which suggests negative feedback, and it is plausible this negative regulation occurs in athletes (normal to high testosterone) and not in infertile men (low testosterone). D-Aspartic Acid causes increases in testosterone synthesis via upregulation of the mRNA that produces a compound called Stimulating Steroidogenic Acute Regulatory Protein which regulates androgen synthesis in the Leydig cells

Improve cognition

Support muscle build[15]

Estrogen metabolism: a 12 week double-blind randomized controlled trial in resistance trained men reported a significant decrease (-16%) in estradiol with 6 g per day supplementation

Dosage

The standard dose for D-Aspartic acid is between 2 to 3g.

Carnitine

The Tartrate form is recognized as being the most natural and well absorbed of the Carnitine family. While acetyl Carnitine is important for brain development, **L-Carnitine tartrate excels at weight loss, heart health and energy creation.** The following are all linked to the benefits of the tartrate form of Carnitine.

Therapeutic Use

Experts say that L Carnitine is it currently the best-researched dietary supplement in the world with 7822 studies listed, and has every appearance of being a proven remedy. Moreover, it is non-toxic, with minimal contraindications and adverse interactions, and well-tolerated by young and old. Whenever an organism needs energy, L-Carnitine plays an important role.

Fat Burning: L-Carnitine mainly increases the rate at which fat is burned. This tends to reduce fat and build up lean muscle mass.[16]

Fatty Acid Transport: L Carnitine is best known as a facilitator of the transport of fatty acids into the mitochondria for oxidation.

Exercise performance: The second lesser known role is in maintaining high density exercise via lactic acid minimalization

Heart Health: Minimizing the risk of heart disease

FYI:

Healthy subjects consumed a high fat meal, which has been shown to cause impairment of vascular health. It was demonstrated in a trial that 2g of L-Carnitine taken with the meal enhanced vascular responses (increased dilation) to the high fat meal. This was most apparent in those subjects who had the greatest decrease in vascular function. Because vascular dysfunction is an early event in heart disease, Carnitine supplementation can be viewed as a preventative or therapeutic supplement to improve risk for heart disease.

Contraindications

The only contraindications for the use of l-Carnitine are to do with specific diseases and conditions.

Seizures: If you have ever had a seizure, you should avoid using l-Carnitine. For people with a history of seizures, the use of L-Carnitine has produced an increase in the seriousness and number of seizures, whether taken intravenously or orally.

Hypothyroidism: if you have an under-active thyroid gland, or hypothyroidism, l-Carnitine tartrate may interact with the hormones produced by the thyroid and could have a negative effect. If you know you have hypothyroidism, it is best to avoid taking additionally l-Carnitine tartrate.

Dosage: 2g: Most studies are done at this dose, taking Carnitine post training. Take with carbs (40-80g) for an insulin spike to help shunt Carnitine into muscle tissue for peak performance.

Acetyl - l-carnitine

Also known as: Acetil-L-Carnitina, Acetyl Carnitine, Acétyl Carnitine, Acetyl L-Carnitine, Acétyl-L-Carnitine, Acetyl-L-Carnitine Arginate Dihydrochloride, Acetyl-L-Carnitine Arginate HCl

Acetyl forms of amino acids are directly taken into the brain, and Carnitine is no exception. The majority of actions take place, with the Acetyl form used to treat **memory related illness and neuropathies.**

The body can convert Acetyl L Carnitine into L Carnitine and vice versa, however, if you are wanting weight loss, best use L Carnitine alone and if you are treating any related brain disorders, use the Acetyl form.

Acetyl L Carnitine is used for age related memory loss, Alzheimer's disease, late life depression, cataracts, pain due to diabetes (type 2) and pain associated with drug that are used to treat AIDS. In relation to **Alzheimer's disease,**[17] this amino acid seems to work best with reducing rapid onset Alzheimer's disease presenting in those under 65 years of age. Also great for muscle function, Acetyl L Carnitine is **vital for the health of the heart muscle and also reduces prostate inflammation**. Useful also for increasing aged related testosterone decline.

Dosages

Alzheimer's disease: 2-4 g in divided doses Age and alcohol related memory loss: 2 g Male Infertility: 1g Acetyl and 2 g L Carnitine. Use an additional 2-5 g L Arginine for sperm motility Age related testosterone deficiency: 2g Acetyl-l-carnitine.

Carnitine Neuropathies: 2-3 g daily

Contraindications: Blood thinners: caution with Warfarin.

Avoid with hypothyroidism.

Side Effects: Nausea, vomiting, "fishy" breath, increased urination and sweating.

Choline

Also known as: Trimethyl-ethanolamine, Choline Bitartrate

Primary Use: Cognitive Function and Brain Health

Other uses: General Health, Liver Health and Detoxification

Choline Bitartrate

In the 1970's, researchers discovered the connection between the precursor choline and acetylcholine.

Choline is a molecule mostly used for either its cognitive boosting properties (turning into acetylcholine, the learning neurotransmitter) or as a liver health agent, able to reduce fatty liver buildup. Found in high amounts in egg, the yolks in particular.

Brain Health: Due to its effect on the brain, choline has been shown to help with symptoms relating to Alzheimer's, dementia, and other age-related memory conditions. Aside from cognitive diseases and conditions, choline is also helpful for **Huntington's, asthma, allergies, Tourette's, and schizophrenia**. Every cell in the human body uses choline to build its outer membrane, which keeps it from being dissolved in the bloodstream.[18]

Acetylcholine transmits electrical impulses from neurons, messenger molecules such as platelet activating factor (PAF), which triggers clotting of blood and activation of the sneezing reflex

Note: The bi-tartrate form of Choline, although being easily absorbed does not so easily cross the blood brain barrier (BBB), such as the acetyl choline form of amino acid. Although some choline bi-tartrate will convert to acetylcholine and make it to the brain, although the primary **role of bi-tartrate is fat loss by lipolysis**, which encourages the use of fat over glucose as the body's primary energy source. It may also be beneficial for the prevention of future weight gain and prevention of fatty liver disease.

Athletes

Many athletes also take choline to help delay fatigue. Athletes that benefit the most are weight lifters and body builders, although endurance athletes also benefit. Choline works best pre exercise as working out will allow this fat to burn at an even faster rate. Choline is an "old school" amino acid to take as a "stack' with carnitine and a small amount of caffeine.

Side effects

Consuming a high amount of choline may cause you to have a fishy body odor, according to the Linus Pauling Institute. Taking an excess of 10 to 16 g a day can cause this undesirable effect and also cause you to sweat and salivate profusely. These conditions are caused by an increased amount of trimethylamine, which is a byproduct of metabolizing choline.

Contraindications

Low blood pressure. Taking more than 7 to 8 g of choline can significantly decrease your blood pressure, leading to hypotension. This can cause dizziness and fainting. Interesting fact:

Choline bi-tartrate provides about 7 times as much choline as the more commonly used phosphatidylcholine supplements and up to 10 times as much choline as lecithin, although as stated, not all crosses the blood brain barrier. Unlike another readily absorbed form of choline, choline magnesium salicylate, choline bitartrate will not cause stomach upset, aspirin allergies, or "tingly" sensations, all of which are cause by the salicylate part of the product, not the choline itself.

Dosage: 1g: I – 3g x a day for weight loss pre exercise and 1g 3 x day for brain health.

Doses for choline vary significantly. Typically, a dose of 250mg to 500mg is used for general health purposes once daily. For mechanisms through acetylcholine, the choline should be pulsed in high doses acutely as higher doses are partitioned to the brain to a greater extent. 1-2g is typically used.

Citrulline

Also known as: L-Citrulline, watermelon extract

Primary Use: Muscle Gain and Exercise

Other uses: Cardiovascular

Available forms: l-Citrulline, DL-Malate

It is turned into L-Arginine in the kidneys after supplementation, which means L-Citrulline supplementation is a more effective method of increasing L-Arginine levels in the body than L-Arginine supplementation.

According to the book, "Nutritional Supplements in Sports and Exercise;" Arginine and Citrulline work together since Arginine also promotes the natural production of Citrulline in your body. A high intake of Arginine causes an increase in blood levels of Citrulline, however large doses of Arginine for vasodilation and NO production may cause unwanted side effects.

Not enough is known about the exact relationship between Arginine and Citrulline to determine the exact dose of Citrulline while also taking Arginine.

Metabolism of Citrulline

You can obtain Citrulline from food, especially watermelons, and it can be also manufactured from Ornithine, in the body's urea cycle. This cycle helps rid your body of ammonia, a waste product of protein digestion. After your digestive system metabolizes Citrulline malate into Citrulline, enzymes in your liver cells convert it into Arginine, then into nitric oxide in a process that also produces new Citrulline molecules. Nitric oxide is a vasodilator that can help protect you from cardiovascular problems by lowering blood pressure and improving blood flow to organs.

Supplementing **L-Citrulline also increases Ornithine and Arginine** plasma content. This means L-Citrulline supplementation improves the ammonia recycling process and nitric oxide metabolism. L-Citrulline is also used to alleviate erectile dysfunction caused by high blood pressure.

Arginine vs Citrulline

L-Arginine and L-Ornithine are subject to reduced absorption when supplemented in doses of 10g or more, which can result in diarrhea. L-Citrulline does not have this side-effect, and since it increases plasma levels of all three amino acids, it may be the preferred as a supplement over L-Arginine. L-Citrulline doubles Ornithine plasma content.

Supplemental L-Arginine provides a spike of L-Arginine in plasma, while supplemental L-Citrulline increases Arginine plasma levels over a longer period of time.

Dosage: **A study published in 2008 by the "British Journal of Nutrition" found that short-term supplementation of Citrulline in 2 to 15 g doses is safe and well-tolerated. Another study published in 2002 by the "British Journal of Sports Medicine" found that 6 g per day of Citrulline supplementation promoted aerobic energy production and changes in muscle metabolism in healthy subjects during exercise.**[19]

To supplement L-Citrulline for circulatory health or to alleviate erectile dysfunction, take 1,000 mg of Citrulline, three times a day with meals, for a total daily dose of 3,000 mg. L-Citrulline does not need to be taken with meals, however. To supplement for circulatory health with a Citrulline malate supplement, take 1.76 g of Citrulline malate for every 1 g of Citrulline you would normally take. To supplement L-Citrulline to enhance sports performance, take 6,000 – 8,000 mg of Citrulline malate about an hour before exercise.

Creatine

Also Known As: Creatine monohydrate, Creatine 2-oxopropanoate, a-methyl-guanidinoacetic acid.

There are many different forms of Creatine available on the market, but Creatine monohydrate is the cheapest and most effective. Another option is micronized Creatine monohydrate, which dissolves in water more easily and can be more practical.

Creatine is a well-researched amino acid predominantly used to **improve exercise performance** by rapidly producing energy during activity. It is often used by athletes to increase both power output and lean mass. It also provides **cognitive benefits.**

It stores high-energy phosphate groups in the form of Phosphocreatine. Phosphocreatine releases energy to **aid cellular function during stress**. This effect causes strength increases after Creatine supplementation, and can also benefit the brain, bones, muscles, and liver. Most of the benefits of Creatine are a result of this mechanism.[20]

Creatine is best **taken with water** as its supplementation may cause cramping in a dehydrated state. Diarrhea and nausea can occur when too much Creatine is supplemented at once, in which case doses should be spread out throughout the day and taken with meals.

Creatine can be found in some foods, mostly meat, egg, and fish. Creatine has neuroprotective and cardioprotective properties.

Do Not Confuse with Creatinine (metabolite), Cyclocreatine (analogue), Creatinol O-phosphate (analogue)

Dosage: Creatine monohydrate can be supplemented through a loading protocol. To start loading, take 0.3 g per kg of bodyweight per day for 5–7 days, then follow with at least 0.03 g/kg/day either for three weeks (if cycling) or indefinitely (without additional loading phases). Higher doses (up to 10 g/day) may be beneficial for people with a high amount of muscle mass and high activity levels or for those who are non-responders to the lower 5 g/day dose.

Cysteine

Also known as: (R)-2-Amino-3-mercaptopropionic acid; beta-Mercaptoalanine; Thioserine; CySH; 3-Mercapto-L-Alanine

Cysteine is a sulphur-containing non-essential amino acid. Cysteine is used to **produce Glutathione** and Taurine. Cysteine is a scavenger of oxidative stress, its most important role is reviving glutathione, one of the most powerful antioxidants in the body. Being a key constituent of glutathione, this amino acid supports a lot of vital physiological functions. Glutathione is made from Cysteine, Glutamic acid, and Glycine, and can be found in all tissues of the human body. Cysteine is essential for the detoxification.

Cysteine is needed for **detoxification** processes in the liver protecting against damage of smoke, alcohol, radiation, toxins and drug on the liver.

Cysteine is a co-enzyme in various enzymatic reactions – redox reactions in which the thiol group protects against peroxidation, and conjugation reactions, in which glutathione in the liver binds with toxic chemicals to detoxify.

Glutathione is needed for detoxification of heavy metals, pesticides, plastics and toxicants for detoxifying effects of Cysteine resulting in increasing Glutathione levels. Useful in baldness, psoriasis, mucus and bronchial congestion. Cysteine enhances effect of topically applied silver, tin, zinc in preventing dental cavities useful in cobalt toxicity, diabetes, psychosis.

Cysteine provides resistance to the body against all harmful effects, because it is responsible for **building up white blood-cell activity**. Cysteine is also necessary for the proper functioning of the skin, recovery of hair and nail tissue and helps the body heal.

Cysteine helps promote **building muscles**, healing of severe burns, reduce the effects of aging **and fat burning.** Cysteine also encourages the activity of white blood cells. L-Cysteine is also valued for its ability to **break up mucus**, thereby making it easier to cough up phlegm that's caused by respiratory and **pulmonary conditions**. L-Cysteine is involved in regulating Glutamate levels, influencing the neurons in the central nervous system.

The activated form, N-acetyl Cysteine has numerous health benefits including its use in bronchitis, angina and acute respiratory distress, liver detoxification and improve immune system functioning.

Cysteine is found in pork, chicken, egg, milk, and cottage cheese. Vegetarians are recommended to consume more garlic, granola and onions.

Dosage: 200–600 mg twice daily.

N-acetyl-Cysteine

Also known as: N-Acetyl Cysteine, NAC

Primary Use: Antioxidant and Anti-inflammatory

Other uses: Liver Health and Detoxification

N Acetyl Cysteine, also known as NAC, an amino acid of the sulfhydryl group, is a precursor of Cysteine and reduced glutathione which enhances the production of Glutathione, a potent anti-oxidant.

N-Acetylcysteine (NAC) is a prodrug for L-Cysteine, which is used for the intention of allowing more glutathione to be produced when it would normally be depleted. Through glutathione buffering, NAC provides anti-oxidative effects and other benefits.

NAC and Liver clearance

Well studied for protecting liver damage from paracetamol overdose, carbon monoxide poisoning, carbon tetrachloride. Inhibits growth of Helicobacter Pylori. Decreases inflammatory cytokines in the gut.

Reduces heavy metal overload: Arsenic, lead, cadmium, mercury, copper excess

Estrogen clearance: NAC removes excess estrogen metabolites (E2) by moving through methoxylation and conjugation pathways

NAC and Mental Health

Studies are ongoing using NAC for Bi Polar disorders and are showing positive results

Used for **Traumatic Brain Injury** with improvements in memory loss, sleep deprivation due to trauma and helps control dizziness

Some chemotherapy treatments reduce cognitive function; supplementing with NAC and Lysine during chemotherapy helps prevent this decline

Help with addictions. NAC normalizes Glutamate in the reward centre of the brain through Cysteine-Glutamate exchanges thereby increasing Glutamate clearance. This results in decreased craving and addictive behavior. After about two weeks of 2,400mg NAC supplementation, cigarette usage appears to be reduced voluntarily by around 25%.[21]

Alzheimer's and Parkinson's disease: NAC helps protect neurons from damage and degeneration

Chronic Obstructive Pulmonary disease, Cystic Fibrosis and IPE (isopropyl ether) can respond to treatment with NAC. NAC for **immunity** and lung diseases. Treatment for the common cold, respiratory congestion and influenza. N-Acetylcysteine may reduce some symptoms of COPD by acting as a mucolytic agent and reducing sputum formation.

Strong evidence for use as a chemo-preventative agent, especially for those at high risk of melanoma[22]

Trichotillomania

Preliminary evidence suggests a 31-45% reduction in hair pulling symptoms in persons with trichotillomania when supplementing with 1,200-2,400mg NAC for twelve weeks.

Sjogren's Syndrome

Reduces Homocysteine levels

Prevent complications from kidney disease

Side Effects and Cautions

May reduce copper levels in the body when using for more than 6 weeks. It is suggested the use of copper supplements when using NAC long term would be beneficial.

The smell of NAC can be offensive to some. Drinking though a straw can help with smell.

Interactions

Nitroglycerine :(used in some instances for heart problems) cannot be used with NAC.

Activated Charcoal: avoid taking NAC at the same time as it nullifies the effect of charcoal.

Dosage: Take on an empty stomach for best results

COPD and other chronic lung conditions: 3 g in divided doses

Acute respiratory infections: 1 g twice daily

Liver clearance and Homocysteine: up to 2g daily

N-acetyl D glucosamine (NAG)

Primary Usage: Bone and joint health

N-acetyl D glucosamine (NAG) is a type of monosaccharide that is also related to glucose and is chemically similar to glucosamine. However, unlike glucose, N-acetyl glucosamine is not really a sugar but belong to a class of compounds called amides, although it is commonly described as a carbohydrate.

NAG occurs naturally in the outer shells of certain insects and shellfish and is synthesized from the reaction between glucosamine and acetic acid. Although NAG can be found in certain cosmetic products where it is used as **an exfoliating and anti-wrinkle agent**, its main use is as a dietary supplement in the treatment of **autoimmune diseases**.

IBS, Crohn's and Colitis

The protective wall of the GIT incorporates N-acetyl glucosamine. NAG shows promise in the treatment of inflammatory bowel disease (a class of conditions that includes Crohn's disease: from impaired innate immunity which is an abnormal immune response to microbial invasion, and for colitis), according to a pilot study published in Alimentary Pharmacology and Therapeutics in 2000. Testing on children with severe Crohn's disease and severe ulcerative colitis were conducted. Researchers found that daily treatment with N-acetyl glucosamine led to a significant improvement in symptoms and a **decrease of inflammation** in damaged soft tissue of the GIT in these children.

Auto Immune disease

A 2011 study from the Journal of Biological Chemistry indicates that N-acetyl glucosamine may help suppress the destructive autoimmune response involved in multiple sclerosis.[23]

As Glucosamine Sulphate and HCL are also currently used in the **treatment of Rheumatoid arthritis,** it would be logical to assume that NAG could be used as it suppresses the auto immune response as well as exerts anti-inflammatory effects.

How it works:

NAG is the more direct route to the important macromolecules such as hyaluronic acid, keratin sulfate and chondroitin sulfate. Unlike the low-molecular glucosamine found in glucosamine sulfate or glucosamine hydrochloride, N-acetyl-D-glucosamine is an advanced molecule that **requires fewer enzymatic steps** before being incorporated into the macromolecules of cartilage.

Given that N-acetyl glucosamine saves the user several biochemical steps involved in the conversion of glucose-6-phosphate to N-acetyl glucosamine, it makes an effective product for the treatment of Crohn's disease.

Tissue biopsies taken from gastrointestinal tracts of Crohn's patients showed decreased glucosamine synthetase activity in the inflamed tissues. Because of the loss of this important structural carbohydrate, the inflamed tissues experience rapid loss of epithelial cells.

Suitable for Diabetics

NAG **does not interfere** with glucose metabolism. Low-molecular glucosamine, as in glucosamine sulfate or glucosamine hydrochloride, has been associated with glucose uptake in patients. This probably occurs because low-molecular-weight glucosamine inhibits glucokinase.

Because N-acetyl-D-glucosamine has its own kinase it is not dependent on glucokinase and does not cause a rise in glucose levels when consumed.

Note on Shellfish allergy

Shellfish allergy is triggered by the meat of seafood and not by their shells. Therefore, shellfish allergy does not involve chitin or N-acetyl glucosamine. This means that those with shellfish allergy, take NAG.

Contra Indications

How safe is N-acetyl glucosamine? The results of current safety studies suggest that N-acetyl glucosamine is very safe. However, N-acetyl glucosamine is not recommended for pregnant and breastfeeding women as well as those who are about to undergo surgery.

It should be used cautiously by patients who also suffer from asthma, bleeding disorders and kidney problems.

N-acetyl glucosamine should not be combined with anticoagulant drug such as warfarin.

Side Effects

None noted.

Dosage: 3-6 g daily in divided doses. NAG dissolves readily and is heat stable, so can be added to hot beverages.

L-Glucosamine HCl

Why use Hydrochloride?

Most literature concentrates on Glucosamine Sulphate, only because this is a more prevalent type of glucosamine on the market. In fact, the hydrochloride form is more concentrated than the sulphate form, approximately 3000 mg of sulphate is equivalent to 1500 mg of hydrochloride, and contains substantially less sodium per effective dose than the sulphate form.

Because glucosamine sulphate is stabilized with sodium chloride (table salt) and can contain as much as 30% sodium, there needs to be consideration for individuals who want to reduce their dietary intake of sodium.

Uses for Glucosamine Hydrochloride

Since glucosamine is a precursor for glycosaminoglycans, which are a **major component of cartilage**, supplemental glucosamine may beneficially influence cartilage structure, and alleviate arthritis. There have been multiple clinical trials testing glucosamine as a potential medical therapy for osteoarthritis, some, but not all results have supported its use.

Glucosamine concentrations in plasma and synovial fluid increase significantly from baseline levels when ingesting Glucosamine hydrochloride and these levels could be biologically advantageous to articular cartilage. In the short term however, the levels are still 10 – 100-fold lower than required to positively affect the cartilage and to build new tissue so treatment needs to be long term to be effective.

The use of Glucosamine Hydrochloride as a therapy for **osteoarthritis** appears safe, but watch side effects listed.

Contra Indications

Warfarin interacts with Glucosamine Hydrochloride.

There are several reports showing that taking glucosamine (with or without chondroitin) increase the effect of warfarin on blood clotting. This can cause bruising and bleeding.

Medications for cancer (Antimitotic chemotherapy) may interact with Glucosamine hydrochloride as medications for cancer work by decreasing how fast cancer cells can copy themselves and it is postulated that glucosamine might increase how fast tumor cells replicate themselves

Dosage: Osteoarthritis: 1.5 -2g daily

Knee pain: 1-1.5g daily.

GABA

Also known as: Gamma-Aminobutyric Acid

Primary Usage: Sleep

Other uses: Mood

GABA is the 'downer' neurotransmitter that counters Glutamate (upper), as the two mediate brain activation in a ying-yang manner. Highly important in the brain, oral ingestion of GABA is complex due to its difficulty in crossing the blood brain barrier.

The Role of GABA in regulating anxiety

Anxiety results from a coordinated activity of numerous brain pathways interacting with different neurotransmitters and being modulated by local and distant synaptic relays. The area in the brain where anxiety is primarily initiated is the Amygdala.

The role of the inhibitory neurotransmitter GABA has long been regarded as central to the regulation of anxiety within this neurotransmitter system and the Amygdala. It is within this target area that drug such as benzodiazepines are activated.

It should be remembered that GABA is not the only neurotransmitter important in the modulation of anxiety responses, many other neurotransmitters have been implicated, including serotonin, oxytocin and corticotropin-releasing hormone (CRH).

The brain circuits in the Amygdala are thought to comprise of inhibitory networks of γ-aminobutyric acid-ergic (GABAergic) interneurons which play a key role in the modulation of anxiety responses both in the normal and pathological state.

Precursors to serotonin in the forms of Tryptophan and 5HTP, increase the action of GABA.[24]

Crossing the BBB

There is little evidence that GABA taken orally will be able to cross the Blood Brain barrier entirely, however a number of studies have shown small amounts readily cross. Studies have shown that the addition of activated B3 may also increase the passage through the BBB.

Brain-Gut connection

As many suffers of anxiety attest to finding relief from their symptoms when taking GABA, could there be an additional involvement via the bidirectional signaling between the brain and Enteric nervous system which is located in the gut? This bidirectional signaling between the brain and the ENS is vital in maintaining homeostasis and even though most research thus far has focused on the signaling from the brain to the gut, an increasing number of studies have explored the influence of the gut's microbiota on the brain.

For example, gut microbiota has been shown to improve mood and reduce anxiety in patients with chronic fatigue. It has been found that certain probiotic strains are able to produce GABA in vivo. Specifically, bacteria from the strains Lactobacillus and Bifidobacterium were effective at increasing GABA concentrations in the enteric nervous system.

HGH and performance

Early studies have proven that GABA in brain tissue not only acts on the Amygdala, but also on **increasing human growth hormone (HGH)**. Using GABA as a supplement can increase performance when weight lifting, increase endurance and help with lean muscle mass.

Did you know?

All sorts of other unexpected thing change GABA activity, for example, the chemicals formed by aging whiskey in oak barrels increase GABA's effect in the brain when the chemicals released from the alcohol as a fragrance and reach the brain via inhalation. The fragrance of Oolong tea has a similar effect, increasing GABA's action as does, to a lesser extent, extracts of green and black tea.

Toxicity

GABA is designated GRAS (generally recognized as safe) by the FDA, and there are no reports of any toxic effects from taking GABA.

Side Effects and interactions

First, as always, be extremely cautious about what to recommend if someone is **pregnant or breast-feeding**. Although there is no data on safety while pregnant or breastfeeding it is wise to be cautious.

It's been reported that high doses can have unexpected effects – some people have found that a high dose actually **increases anxiety**.

High doses can also result in skin flushing, or skin tingling but keeping to doses under 2 g, especially when taken in divided doses, should not cause these problems.

Not recommended for people with **bi-polar disorder or a history of seizures.**

Tryptophan, Tyrosine or GABA?

Generally, if the problem is depression try a serotonin booster instead. If there is a susceptibility to serious depression, be careful with GABA as it can trigger a depressive episode. Indeed, if the presenting complaint is depression or low energy, mood and poor concentration, first try boosting serotonin, (Tryptophan) dopamine (Tyrosine) or using adrenal adaptogens.

Interactions and Cautions

Monitor those on Blood pressure medications when using GABA in case the blood pressure becomes excessively low and watch low blood pressure.

Use SSRI's (Serotonin reuptake inhibitors) with caution as GABA can inhibit serotonin and dopamine in some individuals.

Dosage: Anxiety- 1-2g a day in divided doses. To maximize chances of crossing the BBB, take away from meals with an insulin carrier such as honey or mixed with juice or coconut water as well as with an activated B complex, or preferable activated B3 alone.

Athletic Performance: 2-5g dependent on body weight, with an insulin carrier and activated B3. Take at night for best results.

Glutamine

Also known as: L-Glutamine, L-Glutamic acid 5-amide; 2-Aminoglutaramic acid; L-2-Aminoglutaramidic acid; Glutamic acid amide; Glutamic acid 5-amide; Gamma-glutamine; Levoglutamid; Levoglutamide

Primary Use: Gut Health

Other uses: General Health, Muscle Gain and Exercise

L-Glutamine is the most abundant amino acid naturally fermented at low temperature

Athletic Use:

Glutamine is stored in skeletal muscle along with other sites in the body including the intestine, brain and lung. Not much is written about its use in sports medicine and the idea of Glutamine as a muscle repair agent is not well studied, but is used regardless

Glutamine is used to counter some of the side effects of medical treatments. For example, it is used for **side effects of cancer chemotherapy** including diarrhoea, pain and swelling inside the mouth (mucositis), nerve pain (neuropathy), and muscle and joint pains caused by the cancer drug Taxol.

Glutamine is also used to **protect the immune system** and digestive system in people undergoing radio/chemotherapy for cancer of the esophagus.

Additionally, Glutamine is used for improving recovery after bone marrow transplant or bowel surgery, increasing well-being in people who have suffered traumatic injuries, and preventing infections in critically ill people. After surgery or traumatic injury, nitrogen is necessary to **repair the wounds** and keep the vital organs functioning. About one third of this nitrogen comes from Glutamine.

Some people use Glutamine for **digestive system conditions** such as stomach ulcers, ulcerative colitis, and Crohn's disease.[25]

It is also used for depression, moodiness, irritability, anxiety, insomnia.

People who have HIV can use Glutamine to **prevent weight loss** (HIV wasting) as the body uses more Glutamine than it can replace where there are muscle wasting diseases present

Glutamine is also used for **attention deficit-hyperactivity disorder** (ADHD), a urinary condition called cystinuria, sickle cell anemia, and for alcohol withdrawal support.

Caution

People with kidney disease, liver disease, or Reye syndrome (a rare, sometimes fatal disease affecting children that is generally associated with aspirin use) should not take Glutamine. Some people exhibit signs of excitability and wakefulness when taking Glutamine and could be converting Glutamine to Glutamic acid, which could explain these symptoms.

Dosage: For adults ages 18 and older: Doses of 500mg, 1 - 3 times daily, are generally considered safe and used for general stomach complaints and wound healing

Doses as high as 5 to 15g daily (in divided doses), or sometimes higher, may be prescribed by a health care provider for certain conditions. These include Crohn's and chemotherapy support.

Supplementation of L-Glutamine tends to be dosed at 5 g or above, with higher doses being advised against due to excessive ammonia in serum. The lowest dose found to increase ammonia in serum has been 0.75 g/kg, or approximately 51 g for a 70kg individual.

Glycine

Also known as: 2-Aminoacetic acid, Aminoethanoic acid; Glycocoll; Amino acetic acid

Primary Usage: General Health

Other uses: Anti-aging and longevity, bone and joint health, insulin sensitivity, cardiovascular, sleep, liver health and detoxification.

Glycine is an amino acid and neurotransmitter. It can play both stimulatory and depressant roles in the brain. Supplementation can improve sleep quality.

Athletic Use

Control blood sugar levels and **protect against ATP depletion**, optimizing energy levels.

While too much Glycine in the body can cause fatigue, having the proper amount produces the opposite effect - more energy.

As one of the few amino acids that helps **improve blood-sugar storage**, some experts suggest Glycine may increase energy for endurance activities.[26]

Glycine has been shown to help slow muscle breakdown by supplying Creatine to the muscle cells.

For growth-hormone release, Glycine is reportedly more effective when used with Ornithine, Arginine, Glutamine, Tyrosine, Vitamin B6, niacinamide, zinc, calcium, magnesium, potassium, and/or Vitamin C.

Antacid: Glycine is also used as an antacid agent and is reportedly effective for limiting stomach discomfort. In addition, it may help shuttle toxic substances out of the body.

Prostate: Because the prostate contains considerable amounts of Glycine, this nutrient may help promote prostate health. In fact, one study found that Glycine, taken with Alanine and glutamic acid, reduced the amount of swelling in the prostate tissue.

CNS Function: Glycine is necessary for central nervous system function. Research has shown that this amino acid can help inhibit the neurotransmitters that cause seizure activity, hyperactivity, and manic (bipolar) depression. Glycine can also be converted to another neurotransmitter, Serine, as needed, and may be beneficial in the management of schizophrenia.

Leg Ulcers: When applied as a cream.

Caution

Individuals with kidney or liver disease should not consume Glycine without consulting their doctor. Taking any one glycerol based amino acid supplement can cause a disruption of the citric acid or Krebs cycle, and cause a build-up of nitrogen or ammonia in the body, which makes the liver and kidneys work harder to remove waste.

Clozapine (Clozaril) is used to help treat schizophrenia. Taking Glycine along with clozapine (Clozaril) might decrease the effectiveness of clozapine (Clozaril). It is not clear why this interaction occurs yet. Do not take Glycine if you are taking clozapine (Clozaril).

Dosage: For glycemic and sleep benefits, doses of 3-5 g with meals and before bed, respectively, have been used successfully in clinical research.

Athletic and Other Use: 2-6 g daily

CNS: 4 g daily until desired effect is reached. Some clinical trials with schizophrenic patient's use 40 to 90 g daily (based on .8 g per kg body weight)

Ischemic Stroke: Putting 1 teaspoon Glycine under the tongue may help to limit brain damage caused by an ischemic stroke when started within 6 hours of having the stroke.

Leg ulcers: A cream containing 10 mg of Glycine, 2 mg of L-Cysteine, and 1 mg of DL-Threonine per g of cream has been used. The cream is applied at each wound cleaning and dressing change once daily, every other day, or twice daily as needed.

Inositol

Also known as: MyoInositol, Cyclohexanehexol,1,2,3,4,5,6-cyclohexanehexol

Primary Use: Insulin Sensitivity

Other uses: Women's Health

Forms available: Myo-inositol

Inositol usually refers to Myo-Inositol, a small molecule structurally similar to glucose that is involved in cellular signaling. It appears to be an effective anxiolytic at higher doses, and is quite effective in treating insulin resistance and PCOS with standard doses.

Athletic Performance: Fat Loss, Cholesterol Control, Insulin regulation

Panic disorder: Inositol shows some promise for controlling panic attacks and the fear of public places or open spaces (agoraphobia). One study found that Inositol is as effective as a prescription medication. However, large-scale clinical trials are needed before Inositol effectiveness for panic attacks can be proven.

Obsessive-compulsive disorder (OCD): There is some evidence that people with OCD who receive Inositol by mouth for 6 weeks experience significant improvement.

Polycystic ovary syndrome (PCOS): Taking a particular form of Inositol (isomer D-chiro-Inositol) by mouth seems to lower triglyceride and testosterone levels, modestly decrease blood pressure, and promote ovulation in obese or insulin resistant women with polycystic ovary syndrome. Myo-inositol is thought to be converted to D Chiro Inositol in the body. When using Myo-Inositol for PCOS, the dose should be two-three times higher than using D Chiro Inositol alone. Studies into conception show the myo- form stimulates ovulation better than the D Chiro form.[27] Problems breathing in premature infants known as "acute respiratory distress syndrome" when given intravenously (by IV).

Psoriasis brought on or made worse by lithium drug therapy. Inositol doesn't seem to help psoriasis in people not taking lithium.

FYI: Bipolar disorder: There is some concern that taking too much Inositol might make bipolar disorder worse. There is a report of a man with controlled bipolar disorder being hospitalized with extreme agitation and impulsiveness (mania) after drinking several cans of an energy drink containing Inositol, caffeine, Taurine, and other ingredients (Red Bull Energy Drink) over a period of 4 days. It is not known if this is related to Inositol, caffeine, Taurine, a different ingredient, or a combination of the ingredients.

Dosage: For panic disorder: 12 to 18g per day

For obsessive-compulsive disorder: Inositol 18 g per day. For treating symptoms associated with polycystic ovary syndrome: D-chiro-Inositol 2g per day. For treating lithium-related psoriasis: 6 g daily

For the treatment of polycystic ovarian syndrome (PCOS), myo-Inositol is taken in the range of 200-4,000mg once daily before breakfast

Histidine

Also known as: (S)-4-(2-Amino-2-carboxyethyl)imidazole ; (S)-alpha-Amino-1H-imidazole-4-propanoic acid; L-2-Amino-3-(4-imidazolyl)propionic acid; (2S)-2-azaniumyl-3-(3H-imidazol-4-yl)propanoate

Histidine is a semi-essential amino acid, as adults are normally able to produce an adequate amount of it. However, it is classified as an essential amino acid needed to be taken in the diet. This amino acid is also known for being a precursor of histamine - a compound that is generally released by the immune system cells in an allergic reaction and an important neurotransmitter.

Histidine is involved **in regulation of essential trace elements** like iron, copper, molybdenum, zinc, and manganese. Histidine is also needed in formation of metal-bearing enzymes and compounds, such as the antioxidant super oxide dismutase.

Histidine is required for the **growth and repair of tissues**, red blood cell production, and protecting tissues from damage from radiation and heavy metals. It is especially necessary for the formation of myelin sheaths, which are layers surrounding nerves which enables faster transmission of signals to the brain.

Urocanic acid, produced through Histidine, is a major **absorber of ultraviolet radiation** (UVR). This protects skin cells from damage.

It is also a major component (along with β-Alanine) of carnosine, an important antioxidant that slows the progression of multiple degenerative diseases and reduces plaque build-up in the arteries. It may also help improve muscle performance for high-intensity exercise.

Meanwhile, many toxic stimulates the rapid formation of metallothionein inside the cells of the brain, liver, and kidneys to protect these cells. Metallothionein needs Histidine to protect against mineral-enzyme deficiencies and dysregulations.

Prescription drug such as salicylates and steroids have the potential to lower histamine levels. Folic acid deficiency may increase renal loss of histamine with increased catabolism. Histamine supplementation particularly in diabetic patients has been shown to improve hypoglycemia, hyperlipidemia, oxidation and inflammation.

Sulphur intolerances to foods such as broccoli, onions or garlic coupled with elevated blood plasma L-Cysteine levels will give rise to inactivation of Histidine and iron-dependent enzyme Cysteine dioxygenase.

Histidine is involved in **protecting the skin against UV radiation** and reducing inflammation and oxidative stress. Histidine is the precursor for the production of urocanic acid, a substance that accumulates in human skin cells and absorbs UV radiation. By doing so, urocanic acid protects DNA from being damaged by sunlight and thus has been referred to as a "natural sunscreen"[28]

Histidine is used for **rheumatoid arthritis, allergic diseases, ulcers, and anemia** caused by kidney failure or kidney dialysis.

Carnosine, a Histidine derivative has been shown to reduce fat levels and plaque build-up in the arteries. Histidine and carnosine have shown to reduce elevated blood pressure.

Histidine may reduce inflammation by blocking the production of **inflammatory cytokines**, lower fasting blood glucose levels, **suppress appetite**.

Wilson's disease is a rare genetic disease that causes copper to build up in the organs of the body, particularly the liver. Histidine supplementation may cause accumulated copper in the liver to be flushed out in urine.

Histidine deficiency may have a lot of detrimental effects on the body. Symptoms include dry or scaly skin lesions, reduced hemoglobin and subsequent fatigue, anemia, poor hearing and general feeling of un-wellness.

High amounts of Histidine in the body may result in unwanted side effects like headaches, weakness, fatigue, nausea, anorexia, depression, and memory failure. High histamine levels may be seen in neurological disorders sand in schizophrenia.

Foods high in Histidine include protein-based foods include egg, beef, chicken, pork, fish, soybeans, beans, wheat, maize, quinoa, and rice

Dosage: 8-12 mg/kg per day.

Isoleucine

Also known as: (2S,3S)-alpha-Amino-beta-methyl-n-valeric acid; erythro-L-Isoleucine; L-iso-Leucine; (S)-Isoleucine; 2S,3S-Isoleucine

Isoleucine, an essential BCAA is widely recognized to increase endurance and help heal muscle tissue. Isoleucine may have roles as an anti-catabolic agent (without promoting synthesis) similar to HMB.

The primary function of Isoleucine in the body is to **boost energy** levels and to assist the body in recovering from strenuous physical activity. Isoleucine is an intermediate for its ability to induce muscle protein synthesis (stronger than Valine, but much weaker than Leucine) and is able to significantly increase glucose uptake and the usage of glucose during exercise. Isoleucine does not appear to **promote glycogen re-synthesis** or insulin secretion (anabolic mechanisms of glucose metabolism) but may augment insulin-induced glucose deposition.

Isoleucine is an isomer of Leucine and make up one of three branched-chain amino acids which collectively (Isoleucine, Leucine, and Valine) constitute nearly 70% of all the amino acids in the body's proteins. That is why BCAA's are so important.

Isoleucine potentially has **anti-catabolic actions** at the level of amino acids by reducing the rates of gluconeogenesis.

Isoleucine is involved in hemoglobin synthesis, and **regulation of blood sugar** and energy levels. Isoleucine prevents muscle wasting, promote the tissue repair after injury or surgery and has an anabolic effects on the muscle protein synthesis.

Isoleucine is one of the three branched chain amino acids alongside both Leucine and Valine. Relative to the other two BCAAs. Isoleucine does not promote glycogen synthesis.

Dosage: 48-72mg/kg/day or 3.3-4.9g/day

Leucine

Also known as: L-2-Amino-4-methylpentanoic acid; alpha-Aminoisocaproic acid; L-alpha-Aminoisocaproic acid; alpha-Amino-gamma-methylvaleric acid; (S)-2-Amino-4-methylvaleric acid; 4-Methyl-norvaline

Leucine is an essential amino acid which was discovered in its impure form in cheese back in 1819, and just a year later - in its crystalline form from muscles and wool.

Leucine is the primary BCAA. Supplementing Leucine on its own is still beneficial and may be cheaper than BCAA mixes. Leucine appears to be more effective at promoting **gains in muscle** in people with lower dietary protein intake and in the elderly (who tend to have impaired muscle protein synthesis in response to the diet).

Leucine is an activator of the protein known as mTOR, which then induces muscle protein synthesis. The other two BCAAs, Isoleucine and Valine may also activate mTOR, but are much weaker than Leucine.

B-Hydroxy b-methyl-butyrate (HMB) is a metabolite of the branch chain amino acid Leucine protecting and **repairing muscle tissue**, preserving the structural integrity of muscle cells.[29]

Leucine can stimulate release of Insulin from the pancreas, simulating glucose uptake into the cells.

Leucine helps in **regulate blood-sugar levels**, promotes the growth and the recovery of muscle and bone tissues, and production of growth hormone.

This amino acid is also known for preventing the breakdown of muscle proteins caused by injury or stress. In addition, Leucine may be beneficial for people suffering from phenylketonuria.

Leucine is beneficial for muscle building and **weight loss** as well. Leucine aids in burning fat without burning a muscle by sparing the muscle proteins and leaving them to assist in building and in increasing the muscle gain and mass. Leucine, therefore helps lose more body fat while retaining a more lean muscle mass.

Leucine is found in animal food like fish, chicken, beef, also dairy and egg. Vegetarians will invariably be deficient in Leucine.

Dosage: 2 - 6g range for acute usage.

Lysine

Also known as: L-Lysine; Lysine; 56-87-1; H-Lys-oh; Lysine acid; (S)-Lysine

Primary Use: General Health

Other uses: Allergies and Immunity

Lysine is an amino acid commonly paired with Vitamin C in many supplements. While an essential amino acid it does not hold much promise as a supplement beyond reducing the symptoms of **herpes simplex**.

Athletic performance

Lysine is important for proper growth, and it plays an essential role in the production of Carnitine, and is sometimes taken with the 2:1 Arginine to Ornithine ratio to produce HGH.

Lysine appears to help the body absorb calcium, and it plays an important role in the **formation of collagen**, a substance important for bones and connective tissues including skin, tendon, and cartilage, so may help prevent osteoporosis.

Most people get enough Lysine in their diet, although athletes, vegans who don't eat beans, as well as burn patients may need more.

Some studies have found that taking Lysine on a regular basis may help prevent outbreaks of cold sores and genital herpes. Lysine has **antiviral effects** by blocking the activity or Arginine, which promotes HSV replication. Studies suggest oral Lysine is more effective for preventing an HSV outbreak than it is at reducing the severity and duration of an outbreak. One study found that taking Lysine at the beginning of a herpes outbreak did not reduce symptoms.[30]

Lab studies suggest that Lysine in combination with L-Arginine makes bone building cells more active and enhances production of collagen (possibly by association with HGH?)

Dosage

For adults ages 13 and older: Recommendations are 12 mg/kg/day.

An example of a dose often used during an active herpes flare up is 3 – 9 g per day in divided doses for a short period of time. To prevent recurrences, many people take 2-3 g daily. It should be noted that ingesting supplemental L-Arginine at this time will be counterproductive for this purpose and, if the diet is modified to increase Lysine intake, then L-Arginine should be controlled.

Lysine in the diet is considered safe. High doses have caused gallstones. There have also been reports of renal dysfunction, including Fanconi's syndrome and renal failure.

Use with Lysine may increase the risk of nephrotoxicity.

Methionine

Also known as: L-2-Amino-4-(methylthio)butyric acid; S-Methionine; L-alpha-Amino-gamma-methylmercaptobutyric acid; (S)-2-Amino-4-(methylthio)butanoic acid; L-alpha-Amino-gamma-methylthiobutyric acid; L-gamma-Methylthio-alpha-aminobutyric acid; L-2-Amino-4-methylthiobutanoic acid

Athletic Uses

In addition to its role as a precursor in protein synthesis, L-Methionine participates in a wide range of biochemical reactions, including the production of S-adenosylmethionine (SAM or SAMe), L-Cysteine, glutathione, Taurine and sulphate. Methionine is also a glycogenic amino acid and may participate in the formation of D-glucose and glycogen so may help with energy production and stamina

Liver detoxification: The ability of L-Methionine to reduce the liver-toxic effects of such hepatotoxins as acetaminophen and methotrexate has led to the suggestion that Methionine should be added to acetaminophen products. However, there is some recent research suggesting that elevated L-Methionine intake may promote intestinal carcinogenesis. This is unclear.[31]

Heavy Metal Toxicity: L-Methionine is involved in the formation of many substances containing protein, as well as providing sulphur. It is necessary for the bonding and excretion of toxic heavy metal compounds.

UTI's: Methionine is also capable of pushing the pH-value of urine into the acidic part of the scale, reducing the occurrence of cystitis and other urinary tract infections. The effectiveness and efficiency of ampicillin and other antibiotics is also improved where the pH-value ranges between 4 and 6.

Absorption

L-Methionine is metabolized in the intestines and transported to the liver for protein biosynthesis. Methionine is involved in a wide variety of metabolic reactions, including the formation of SAMe,

L-Homocysteine, L-Cysteine, Taurine and sulphate. There is where it is also metabolized to produce D-glucose and glycogen.

Cautions and Interactions

One of the metabolites of L-Methionine, L-Homocysteine, has been implicated as a significant factor in coronary heart disease and other vascular diseases. Perhaps taking Methionine with Taurine, B6, B12 & Folate may counter this production?

Methionine, Creatine and SAMe may inhibit absorption of L-Dopa, Parkinson's medication.

Methionine as a methylation cofactor and precursor is best taken with B-complex vitamins, particularly vitamin B6, vitamin B12 and folate as Methionine may increase blood levels of Homocysteine and cholesterol, both of which are linked to elevated risks for atherosclerosis.

Dosage: 2g per day

Even without B-vitamin deficiencies, taking high doses of Methionine 7g daily or more can increase Homocysteine levels.

Ornithine

Also known as: L-Ornithine

Primary Usage: Muscle Gain and Exercise

Ornithine is one of the three amino acids involved in the Urea cycle, alongside L-Arginine and L-Citrulline; this amino acids appears to reduce elevated ammonia levels when supplemented, and preliminary evidence suggests an ergogenic role due to this.

Athletic Performance

Stimulation of HGH in combination with Arginine HCL. L-Ornithine has an anti-fatigue effect in increasing the efficiency of energy consumption.[32]

Ornithine is the driving force of action of the enzyme Arginase which creates Urea. Therefore, Ornithine is a central part of the urea cycle, which allows for the excess nitrogen and ammonia.

Ornithine uses Ammonia and Nitrogen to produce urea which is then excreted by the kidney.

Used in **Parasite Cleansing** to mop up ammonia produced from parasites. Excessive ammonia can cause insomnia, according to Hulda Clarke.

Possibly an adjunct treat ammonia and nitrogen (shown in blood tests)

Useful for **wound healing**, post-surgery due to the fact that it acts as a precursor of Citrulline, Proline and glutamic acid, all of which play a role in healing.

Interesting Note: High ammonia levels can occur for a variety of reasons ammonia in your blood include parasites, liver failure, hepatitis, liver cirrhosis, Reye's syndrome in children, intestinal bleeding, cardiovascular conditions, kidney complications and a rare, inherited disorder of the urea cycle called Citrullinemia. If left untreated, these conditions can lead to complications like a liver abscess.

Early symptoms of high ammonia levels can include lethargy, confusion, and memory difficulties.

Dosage: Parasites: 1-3 g at night

Athletes: 3-6 g. L Ornithine HCl is generally considered safe to take in high doses.

Ornithine supplementation (as hydrochloride) is taken in the range of 2-6g daily.

There is a chance of intestinal distress at doses above 10g.

Phenylalanine

Also known as: L-beta-Phenylalanine; L-2-Amino-3-phenylpropionic acid; (S)-alpha-Amino-benzenepropanoic acid; (S)-alpha-Aminohydrocinnamic acid; (S)-alpha-Amino-beta-phenylpropionic acid; Phenyl-alpha-Alanine; (-)-beta-Phenylalanine; beta-Phenyl-alpha-Alanine; beta-Phenyl-L-Alanine; 3-Phenyl-L-Alanine; L-beta-Phenylalanine; (S)-Phenylalanine; 3-Phenylalanine

Phenylalanine is found in 3 forms: L-Phenylalanine, the natural form found in proteins; D-Phenylalanine (a mirror image of L-Phenylalanine that is made in a laboratory), and DL-Phenylalanine, a combination of the 2 forms.

Metabolism: L-Phenylalanine acts primarily on the digestive system and the metabolic rate.

One of Phenylalanine's primary functions is to serve as a precursor to the amino acid Tyrosine, which in turn is needed to produce the hormone thyroxine.

Appetite Suppression: Phenylalanine also stimulates the release of cholecystokinin, a digestive system hormone that produces a feeling of satiety after eating and decreases interest in eating, as well as being a precursor molecule for the neurotransmitter noradrenaline, a compound that also plays a role in controlling appetite.

Depression: The body changes Phenylalanine into Tyrosine, which makes proteins, brain chemicals, including L-dopa, adrenaline, and noradrenaline, and thyroid hormones.

Pain Control: D Phenylalanine (but not L-Phenylalanine) has been used to treat chronic pain.[33]

Skin Conditions: Phenylalanine is a precursor to melanin via L Tyrosine so is used in the treatment of Vitiligo along with sunlight therapy.

Cautions: Monoamine Oxidase Inhibitors: Monoamine oxidase inhibitors (MAOIs) are an older class of antidepressants drug that are rarely used now. They include phenelzine (Nardil), isocarboxazid, and tranylcypromine sulfate (Parnate). Taking Phenylalanine while taking MAOIs may cause a severe increase in blood pressure (hypertensive crisis).

Levodopa: A few case reports suggest that Phenylalanine may reduce the effectiveness of levodopa (Sinemet), a medication used to treat Parkinson's disease.

Antipsychotic drug can interact with Phenylalanine. These include chlorpromazine, clozapine, fluphenazine, haloperidol, olanzapine, perphenazine, prochlorperazine, quetiapine, risperidone, thioridazine, thiothixene and others.

Melanoma patients should avoid taking L-Phenylalanine and L-Tyrosine. Certain cancers, such as melanoma, depend on these amino acids to fuel their growth.

Supplemental use of L-Phenylalanine and L-Tyrosine may raise or normalize blood pressure.

Insomnia may be a side effect if taken too close to bedtime.

Some researchers think L-Phenylalanine use can cause a number of side effects, including high blood pressure, nausea, heartburn, difficulty sleeping and mood swing, especially irritability. This is usually due to high dosing.

Dosage: 5g a day for any conditions.

More than 5g can cause neuropathies.

D, L-Phenylalanine competes with other amino acids. They have to be able to pass through the stomach and blood brain barrier without competition. Take Phenylalanine on an empty stomach 15-20 minutes before eating. It is recommended to start with 500-1,000 mg as soon as you awake. Some people may take another 500-1,000 mg 4-6 hours later.

Taking Phenylalanine too close to bedtime may keep you awake.

Proline

Also known as: 2-Pyrrolidinecarboxylic acid; (S)-Pyrrolidine-2-carboxylic acid

Proline is the amino acid necessary for the production of collagen and cartilage for healthy joints, ligaments and skin.

L-Proline for Cardiovascular Health

L-Lysine and particularly L-Proline are important substrates for the biosynthesis of matrix protein and competitively inhibit the binding of lipoprotein to the vascular matrix which prevents cholesterol build up and resulting arterial plaque. Maintaining the integrity and physiological function of the vascular wall is the key therapeutic target in controlling cardiovascular disease.

L-Proline for fine lines and wrinkles

When Proline is taken, the stability of collagen is increased, making it a desirable supplement for skin integrity and decreasing fine lines and wrinkles

L-Proline to heal wounds and collagen synthesis

Proline initiates the biochemical pathway for connective tissue repair and collagen production, therefore increases wound healing and minimizes scar formation.[34]

Dosage:

Reducing cholesterol plaque - Vit C 3 g, Lysine 2 g, Proline 2 g

Skin and wound healing: 2 – 5 g daily, weight dependent

Cautions:

The intake of L-Proline may lead to the development of neurological problems such as seizures and intellectual disability in patients with **hyper-prolinemia**, a rare genetic condition caused by the excesses in Proline levels, according to the Genetics Home Reference of the National Institutes of Health.

If you have high levels of **lactic acid** in your blood, you are also predisposed to hyper-prolinemia, because lactic acid inhibits the breakdown of Proline. People who have **chronic kidney failure** should not take any amino acid supplement without consultation with their physician

Smokers should avoid Proline supplements and foods that are high in Proline if they eat foods preserved with nitrates or that release nitrates during the process of pickling, because, in smokers, nitrates can convert Proline into the potent carcinogen N-nitrosoproline.

People who have **alcohol-related liver disease** should not take Proline, as they usually already have high levels of Proline in the bloodstream.

Chronic liver inflammation interferes with the body's ability to make collagen anywhere except in the liver, where Proline is used to form the collagen that forms the fibers that cause cirrhosis of the liver.

People who have **allergies** should avoid Proline as it increases levels of histamine in the bloodstream.

Serine

Also known as: beta-Hydroxyalanine; (S)-Serine

Serine, a non-essential amino acid, is the precursor to a number of amino acids like Glycine and Cysteine.

D-Serine is an amino acid that plays a role in cognitive enhancement and schizophrenia treatment. D-Serine is an amino acid found in the brain. Derived from Glycine, d-Serine is a **neuromodulator**, meaning it regulates the activities of neurons.

Serine plays an important role in various biosynthetic pathways, helps catalyze hydrolysis of peptide bonds in polypeptides and proteins, which is basically a major function in the **digestive process.**

Serine plays a vital role in **formation of phospholipids** necessary for cell development. In addition, this amino acid is involved in the functioning of RNA and DNA, in the **muscle formation** as well as in the maintenance of a proper immune system. Tryptophan, an essential amino acid **used to make serotonin** (a mood-determining brain chemical), also cannot be produced without Serine. Meanwhile, both serotonin and Tryptophan shortages are believed to cause depression, insomnia, and anxiety. Serine together with Glycine has been shown to improve sleep maintenance without side effects of sleep medications.[35]

Serine is also known for assisting in used in **motor neurone disease, chronic fatigue syndrome and fibromyalgia**, production of immunoglobulins and antibodies for a healthy immune system, as well as for helping in the absorption of Creatine that helps build and maintain the muscles. Vitamin B and folic acid are needed for production of Serine in the body. Naturally, this amino acid can be derived from meat and soy foods, from dairy products, and from peanuts.

Serine supplementation can reduce symptoms of **cognitive decline**.[36]

It is also able to reduce symptoms of diseases characterized by reduced N-methyl-D-aspartate (NMDA) signaling, which includes **cocaine dependence and schizophrenia**. Preliminary evidence suggests that doubling or quadrupling the dosage to 60mg/kg and 120mg/kg, respectively, will cause additional benefits for people suffering from schizophrenia. D-Serine is often categorized as a **nootropic.**

The usual dose used in D-Serine studies is 30mg/kg of bodyweight. This correlates to an approximate dosage range of 2,045 – 2,727mg for people between 70-80kg. This dose appears to be the minimal effective dose for improving cognition in people suffering from a variety of diseases.

Do Not Confuse with Glycine or Sarcosine (similar in mechanisms), Phosphatidylserine

Phosphatidylserine (a phospholipid containing L-Serine) is an amino acid derivative compound that is fat-soluble and found in high amounts in the brain, where it contributes to cognitive functioning. Found in high amounts in fish, it may improve memory in the elderly and lowers cortisol.

Dose: L-Serine- 400-600 mg/kg/day in four to six doses.

Taurine

Also known as: 2-aminoethane sulphonic acid, L-Taurine

Primary Usage: General Health

Other uses: Antioxidant and Anti-inflammatory, Cardiovascular

Taurine is an organic acid containing Sulphur. It is found in foods, in highest amounts in meats, and is a heart and blood healthy agent that can confer a wide variety of health benefits. Its most well-known usage is to reduce cramping caused by fat burners like adrenaline.

Athletic Performance: The amino acid Taurine is believed to enhance the effect of adrenalin in the body by increasing the number of adrenalin receptors in the body, but not enough studies verify this.

The levels of some amino acids can rise in the muscle cells when taking Taurine, specifically Glutamine and the BCAAs Valine, Leucine and Isoleucine. It may be that Taurine raises the concentration function of glycogen precursors.

In a recent study, scientists discovered that Taurine supplements may help **reduce levels of Homocysteine.**

Taurine also occurs naturally in the body and plays a key role in many biological processes, such as **detoxification and regulation of nerve-cell activity**. Although low levels of Taurine have been linked to several conditions (including eye diseases and cardiovascular problems), research on the health benefits of Taurine supplements is fairly limited.

There's some evidence that Taurine may protect against **diabetes** and diabetes-related complications and may help prevent the onset of type 2 diabetes.

Published in Diabetes/Metabolism Research and Reviews in 2001, an earlier report indicates that Taurine supplementation shows promise in the prevention of certain diabetes-related complications (such as atherosclerosis).[37]

Taurine may help treat **high blood pressure**, according to a 2002 report published in Amino Acids. Looking at data from preliminary research, the report's authors found that Taurine supplementation may lead to significant decreases in blood pressure.[38]

Relieving panic attacks and anxiety due to GABA effects of Taurine. Taurine has been shown to be an effective adjunct as an anti-depressant and sedative.[39]

Dosage:

3-5g for panic attacks, anxiety

3-5g for Homocysteine and heart (studies done on 3g for 4 weeks)

6g for athletes (in divided doses) for short periods of time.

The upper limit for toxicity is placed at a much greater level and high doses are well-tolerated. The upper limit for which one can be relatively assured no side effects will occur over a lifetime has been suggested to be 3g a day.

L-Theanine

Also known as: L-Theanine, 5-N-Ethyl-Glutamine

Primary Usage: Mood

L-Theanine is one of the main active ingredients **found in green tea**, alongside caffeine and green tea catechins. It helps promote relaxation without drowsiness, making it synergistic with caffeine.

L-Theanine is an amino acid that is not typically found in the diet and additionally, is not one of the essential amino acids or one of the common nonessential amino acids, however is unique to green tea and certain mushroom species. L Theanine, therefore, is deemed a non-dietary amino acid similar to Ornithine or Citrulline.

The molecular structure of Theanine is similar to Glutamine and **produces the neurotransmitters GABA and Glutamate.**

Theanine, in the brain **acts on the Glutamate transporter**, where, in the neurons, it converts to Glutamine with the assistance of the enzyme glutaminase. L Theanine then is decarboxylated into γ-amino butyric acid (GABA) which also occurs within the neurons. This indicates that L Theanine **modulates GABA** production from Glutamine in the brain. Theanine molecules are small enough to pass through the blood-brain barrier in around half an hour which is why some people prefer L Theanine over GABA which has a poorer BBB passage rate.

Nervous system disorders: The properties of L-Theanine can be summed up as being a **relaxing agent** without sedation, and studies have also shown it reduces the perception of stress and slightly **improves attention.** While L-Theanine does not appear to induce sleep, it may assist with sleep maintenance although it is not recommended on its own as first line treatment for insomnia.

L-Theanine is known to block the binding of L-glutamic acid to Glutamate receptors in the brain. This characteristic of L-Theanine suggests that it may influence psychological and physiological states under **stress.**[40]

L-Theanine has an interesting supplemental role in attenuating the 'edge' of many stimulants. A combination of L-Theanine with caffeine (200mg each) synergistic in **promoting cognition and attention**.

Thermogenesis: L-Theanine may assist in regulating thermogenesis and liver detoxification

Safety, Cautions and Side Effects

L-Theanine is GRAS (generally regarded as safe)

Caution: Theanine recommended to be taken by those who are generally highly anxious, but

not suited to those who are in an inhibitory state, or if someone presents with low serotonin levels. While small amounts of

L-Theanine won't affect most users, a dosage of 1500 mg or more a day may reduce serotonin, potentially causing side effects including brain fog, depression, and low energy. Dizziness, nausea, and headaches are a common side effect evident in clinical studies of L-Theanine.

Reduced appetite is another, sometimes welcomed, side effect!

Contraindications

Low Serotonin, SSRI medications

Pseudoephedrine, adrenaline and other stimulant drug may be decreased in effectiveness when taken with L Theanine

Dosage: 300mg-500 mg taken in water or juice away from meals, preferably in divided doses. May also be taken with caffeinated beverages.

L-Theanine tends to be taken in the dosage of 100-200mg, usually alongside caffeine

Threonine

Also known as: L-Theanine, (2S,3R)-2-Amino-3-hydroxybutyric acid; L-2-Amino-3-hydroxybutyric acid; (S)-Threonine

Primary use: depression, liver detoxification

Athletic use: May speed wound healing and recovery from injury by keeping the connective tissue strong to facilitate faster healing. Threonine is needed to **create Glycine and Serine**, two amino acids that are necessary for the **production of collagen, elastin, and muscle tissue.**

It is also found in significant amounts in the heart.

Liver Function: Threonine combines with the amino acids Aspartic acid and Methionine to help the liver with the digestion of fats and fatty acids.

Nervous System Disorders: Threonine supplementation may be useful in the treatment of Lou Gehrig's disease, Amyotrophic

Lateral Sclerosis (ALS) where there is a Glycine deficiency. Administering Glycine directly is ineffective, since it cannot cross into the central nervous system, so it needs Threonine to facilitate the shuttle. Research indicates that symptoms of Multiple Sclerosis (MS), another disease that affects the nerve and muscle function, may be lessened with Threonine supplementation.

Uric acid reduction: Uric acid accumulation in the body predisposes the body to Gout. The amino acid Threonine, along with Glycine, are important compound for the removal of purines - these are compounds that break down into uric acid, which itself is a by-product of protein digestion in the human body.

Dosage

When taken in dosage of anything between 2 and 4 g every day for a maximum period of about 12 months the use of Threonine appears to be safe. However, some people using this essential amino acid may suffer from negligible side effects like headache, stomach disorder, queasiness and skin rash.

Nervous System Disorders: ALS, MS, Depression

One 1992 study showed that 7.5 g of Threonine taken daily decreased spasticity among study participants. Individuals suffering from clinical depression can also benefit from using dosages consisting of one g of Threonine two times daily - this supplementation generates a marked improvement in the affected person.[41]

Tryptophan

Also known as: L-Tryptophan, TRP; 2-Amino-3-(1H-indol-3-yl)propanoic acid; (S)-2-Amino-3-(3-indolyl)propionic acid; L- alpha-Amino-3-indolepropionic acid; alpha'-Amino-3-indolepropionic acid; Indole-3-Alanine; Indole-3-propionic acid, alpha-amino-; 1-beta-3-IndolylAlanine; Propionic acid

Primary Usage: Fat Loss, depression

Other uses: Mood, depression, glucose tolerance

Tryptophan is an essential amino acid. It is the **precursor to 5-hydroxytrypophan** (5-HTP) which is the direct precursor to serotonin. Serotonin is important for mood and sleep; when it is deficient, this can lead to anxiety, depression, insomnia, and various other neuropsychological conditions. L-Tryptophan is naturally fermented at low temperature.

L Tryptophan works in about 50% of insomnia cases.[42]

Tryptophan is the **precursor for vitamin B3** in the form of nicotinamide adenine dinucleotide (NAD). Only about 1/60th of the Tryptophan in the body is actually converted to NAD.

Tryptophan is useful for:

Mood: Mood disorders, PMT, sleep and other conditions directly affected by reduced Serotonin production and uptake.

Skin: Because it is a precursor to B3, Tryptophan may also be useful for dermatitis and pellagra.

Weight loss: Tryptophan decreases carbohydrate craving, and, because of its ability to convert into B3, helps with the metabolism of fats, carbohydrates and proteins condition called cystinuria, sickle cell anemia, and for alcohol withdrawal support.

Absorption into the Brain: The brain typically receives less than one percent of ingested Tryptophan. However, getting even this small share of Tryptophan is a difficult task for the brain, due to the blood brain barrier (BBB). The BBB makes it hard even for brain essential nutrients to enter the brain. Serotonin by itself cannot penetrate the BBB, but its precursor, Tryptophan, can. Nutrients must be ferried through the BBB by transport molecules, and unfortunately for the serotonin-using nerves, Tryptophan must share its transportation route with five other amino acids: Tyrosine, Phenylalanine, Valine, Leucine and Isoleucine. Taking a supplement therefore, increases the chance of uptake into the brain which food alone may not be able to achieve.

Heat sensitivity and solubility: Tryptophan is heat sensitive and losses in cooking range from between 65% in pork and 46%

in chicken that have been cooked by either frying, roasting or grilling. Therefore, it is wise not to mix Tryptophan powder in with very hot water.

This is unfortunate as Tryptophan can have solubility issues, but this can be resolved by being vigilant in using heated water or encapsulating the product. Using Tryptophan as a powder is preferable, however it has a very light molecular weight of 1g per 5ml teaspoon.

Beware Serotonin Syndrome: This is where there is an excess Tryptophan or 5-HTP levels, usually as a result with prescription anti-depressants. Signs and symptoms include agitation, confusion, delirium, tachycardia and blood pressure changes.

Cautions:

Fluoxetine and Related **Selective Serotonin Reuptake Inhibitor** and Serotonin-Noradrenaline Reuptake Inhibitor (SSRI and SNRI) Antidepressants – Additive effect can result in rapid onset of severe symptoms but might also be applied purposefully within a tightly managed therapeutic protocol. Generally, avoid concomitant use or under close supervision with a healthcare professional.

Phenelzine and Related **Monoamine Oxidase Inhibitors** – Concomitant use carries high probability of resulting in clinically significant serotonin excess and major risk of serious adverse effects. Avoid concomitant use.

Sibutramine and other **Serotonin Agonists** – Concomitant use can lead to clinically significant serotonin excess and major risk of serious adverse effects. Avoid concomitant use.

Tricyclic Antidepressants – Tryptophan can increase the action of TCAs. This additive effect can result in rapid onset of severe symptoms but might also be applied purposefully within a tightly managed therapeutic protocol.

Contraindications: Achlorhydria, bladder cancer, diabetes mellitus, female infertility, psoriasis.

Possible side effects: Anorexia, dizziness, headaches, dry mouth, nausea

Dosage:

Anxiety, Depression and PMT: 2-6 g in divided doses in capsule form or in water between meals. Take with a small amount of carbohydrate to shuttle into the blood brain barrier.

Weight loss and skin: 1-2g in water between meals. Take with a small of carbohydrate to shuttle into cells.

Insomnia: 1-3g 1 hour before bed with a small amount of carbohydrate Although studies show Tryptophan is safe up to 15g, stick to maximum dose of 6 g to prevent serotonin syndrome

Although studies show Tryptophan is safe up to 15g, aim at a dose of 6g daily to prevent Serotonin Syndrome.

Tyrosine

Also known as: 3-(4-Hydroxyphenyl)-L-Alanine; (S)-alpha-Amino-4-hydroxy-benzene-propanoic acid; (-)-alpha-Amino-p-hydroxyhydrocinnamic acid; L-p-Tyrosine; p-Tyrosine; (S)-Tyrosine;L-Beta-(p-Hydroxyphenyl)Alanine;(S)-alpha-Amino-hydroxybenzenepropanoic acid

Primary Usage: Mood

L-Tyrosine is an amino acid that is used to produce noradrenaline and dopamine; supplemental appears to be anti-stress for acute stressors (which tend to deplete noradrenaline) and may preserve stress-induced memory deficits.

Athletic Use: Supplements that boost the brain's dopamine concentration are of interest to endurance athletes. Some research has suggested that Tyrosine might have an effect at a high temperature.

At high temperatures athletes tire more quickly. In the brain Tyrosine is converted – also via L-Dopa – into dopamine. Dopamine is a neurotransmitter that motivates people to continue and suppresses feeling of fatigue and is **activated by high temperatures produced by aerobic activity.**

Cognitive function

Tyrosine supplements helped protect against the detrimental effects of severe cold exposure on cognitive performance and memory. The main effects of L-Tyrosine that have been reported are acute effects in preventing a decline in cognitive function in response to physical stress.[43]

Depression and mood disorders

Tyrosine (actually L-Tyrosine) is an amino acid precursor of the neurotransmitters nordrenaline and dopamine. Taking Tyrosine on an empty stomach is supposed to cause an increase in noradrenaline and dopamine in the brain, which can lead to increased energy, alertness and improved moods, thus relieving depression.

Unlike St John's wort, that can take two months to work, and prescription antidepressants, which probably won't kick in for about six weeks, **Tyrosine works very quickly**.

However, because it **can raise blood pressure** in some people, it must be used cautiously by individuals with hypertension and can also cause anxiety.

Healing the thyroid can be a useful adjunct in the treatment of depression. As a precursor of the thyroid hormones thyroxine and tri-idothyronine, L Tyrosine can help to **elevate mood** and promote well-being that is hindered by low thyroid function.

PKU (phenylketonuria): This serious condition occurs in people whose bodies can't use the amino acid Phenylalanine. It can lead to brain damage, including intellectual disability.

People with PKU must avoid any Phenylalanine in their diets. Because Tyrosine is made from Phenylalanine, people with PKU can be deficient in Tyrosine.

Dosage:

Thyroid Function and Mood disorders 500-1000 mg twice daily

PKU: 500-1000mg once daily

Take L Tyrosine at least 30 minutes before meals, divided into 2-3 daily doses.

L-Tyrosine tends to be taken in doses of 500-2000mg approximately 30-60 minutes before any acute stressor such as extreme exercise.

Taking vitamins B6, B9 (folate), and copper along with Tyrosine helps the body convert Tyrosine into important brain chemicals. There is no research to indicate taking Tyrosine in juice enhances absorption.

Cautions: Monoamine Oxidase Inhibitors (MAOIs) - Tyrosine may cause a severe increase in blood pressure in people taking antidepressant medications known as MAOIs.

This rapid increase in blood pressure, also called "hypertensive crisis," can lead to a heart attack or stroke. People taking MAOIs should avoid foods and supplements containing Tyrosine.

MAOIs include Isocarboxazid, Phenelzine, Tranylcypromine, Selegiline

Thyroid hormones -Tyrosine is a precursor to thyroid hormone, so it might raise levels too high when taken with synthetic thyroid hormones.

Levodopa (L-dopa) - Tyrosine should not be taken at the same time as levodopa, a medication used to treat Parkinson's disease. Levodopa may interfere with the absorption of Tyrosine.

Valine

Also known as: L-2-Amino-3-methylbutyric acid; (S)-α-Amino-isovaleric acid; L-alpha-Amino-isovaleric acid

Valine is one of the three **branched chain amino acids**, although infrequently tested in isolation and possibly the least important BCAA for body composition and does not appear to have any known unique benefits associated with it.

It seems to be more **similar to Leucine** than it is to Isoleucine, but the transient state of insulin resistance occurs faster than with Leucine (Isoleucine causes glucose uptake) while the **muscle building effects** of Valine are likely less than both Leucine and Isoleucine.

Valine provides numerous benefits like improvement in **insomnia and nervousness**. Besides, it is also proved to help alleviate disorders of the muscles, and to be an effective **appetite suppressant.**

This amino acid also greatly improves the regulation of the **immune system,** but probably the greatest benefits of Valine are experienced by athletes performing long-distance sports and **bodybuilding**, because this amino acid is important for the **muscle tissue recovery** and for the muscle metabolism, while increasing exercise endurance.

Bodybuilders and athletes usually use Valine together with Isoleucine and Leucine (BCAA) to promote muscle growth and to supply them with an energy, muscle metabolism and the growth of muscle tissue.

Valine prevents the breakdown of muscle supplying muscles with glucose responsible for energy production during physical activity. Valine is also a precursor in the penicillin biosynthetic pathway and is known for inhibiting the transport of Tryptophan across the blood-brain barrier.

Valine has been noted to increase insulin secretion from the pancreas, but is approximately 3-9% (health persons and those with impaired glucose tolerance) as potent as glucose itself and weaker than L-Arginine (46-61%), but in type II diabetics increases to 47% (Arginine at 180%).[44]

Valine is an essential amino acid important for smooth **nervous system** and **cognitive functioning**. Valine is one of the three branched-chain amino acids, along with Leucine and Isoleucine.

This amino acid cannot be produced by your body and must be obtained through food or through supplements. Valine is important for everyday body functions and for **maintaining muscles**, as well as for the regulation of the **immune system**. This particular amino acid is not processed by the liver, but is taken up by muscles.

Valine is found in kidney beans, leafy vegetables, poultry and milk.

Therapeutic Value of Amino Acids

Amino Acids are used therapeutically in medicine. Think about it, almost all enzymes that catalyze biochemical reactions in the body, plasma proteins carrying minerals and hormones to target tissues or gene markers that control our familial traits are in fact, amino acids.

Liver function tests involve measure of amino acid transaminase enzymes such as Alanine transaminase (ALT) Aspartate transaminase (AST).

The CBS, cystathionine beta-synthase is a gene containing an amino acid component responsible for using vitamin B6 to convert Homocysteine and Serine to cytathionine.

Plasma proteins like albumin, fibrinogen, prothrombin, and the gamma globulins are involved in maintenance of osmotic pressure, transporting lipids and steroid hormones to target tissues.

The therapeutic value of amino acids requires a deeper understanding of each amino acid in respect **essentiality** or classification to identify whether it needs to be derived from the diet or to supplement.

Histadine and Tryptophan, for example must come from the diet. If the diet is insufficient of protein, these amino acids required to synthesize Histamine and Serotonin will be deficient manifesting as depression or neurological imbalances.

Therapeutic nature of amino acids determines its physiological action in the body.

Cysteine, Taurine and Methionine are Sulphur-containing amino acids required for sulphation conjugation in phase 2 liver detoxification.

Synthesis and Metabolism

Most amino acids are derived from other amino acids or metabolized to amino acids for its therapeutic role.

Serine is an intermediary precursor of Glycine needed in synthesis of GABA.

Both Serine and Glycine have their own properties and functions but are connected through synthesis.

Utilization of amino acids

The use of amino acids in the body is highly tissue and time-dependent. During sleep, for example the rate of melatonin synthesis increases and many tissues actively removing amino acids from the blood for tissue repair, neuronal plasticity and detoxification. Cortisol rises in the morning and amino acids are broken down from skeletal muscle and oxidized for energy.

During the allergy season, gastric mucosal cells and mast cells have a larger demand for histamine to supply for the formation of histamine.

Tryptophan demand by the intestine is increased during gastrointestinal discomfort, diarrhea where serotonergic cells in the brain increase utilization of Tryptophan. In conditions of IBS or IBD, gastrointestinal mucosal cells are the largest consumers of Tryptophan for serotonin synthesis but may be diminished in conditions of inflammation of the gastrointestinal tract.

Amino acids influence practically every metabolic pathway in the body. I will highlight the **key therapeutic roles of amino acids**.

For more detailed information, please see **Alchemy of Amino Acids Online Masterclass**.

Regulation of acid base balance

When amino acids are degraded in the liver, glutamic acid is produced and then nitrogen or ammonia is transformed into urea via the urea cycle. Glutamate carries nitrogen away from exercising muscle via alpha ketoglutarate. Glutamine is involved in detoxification of ammonia.

Glutamine and Glycine regulate systemic pH in the kidney, liver and brain during food intake. Academia is associated with low Glutamine.

The net effect of acidosis is to increase the flow of Glutamine from the liver to the kidney where the ammonia is removed, thereby lowering systemic pH.

Acidosis stimulates Glutamine uptake in the kidney, tending to produce a low plasma Glutamine. Low or high Glutamate and Glutamine is found in chronic headaches, fibromyalgia pain or infectious diseases.

Acidosis is associated with low Glutamine. The net effect of acidosis is an increase in flow of Glutamine from the liver to the kidney where the ammonia is removed, thereby lowering systemic pH.

Acidosis stimulates Glutamine uptake in the kidney, tending to produce a lower plasma Glutamine. Low or high Glutamate and Glutamine is found in chronic headaches, fibromyalgia pain or infectious diseases.

Amino acids in exercise and sport Nutrition

Protein powders of frequently used by athletes in exercise and sport industries to improve muscle mass and gain strength. Essential amino acid intake has an immediate effect of reducing muscle protein breakdown and release of muscle amino acids into plasma.

Three reasons why amino acids are beneficial for exercise:

1.Build energy supply

BCAA intake prior to a workout will prime the body to provide sufficient energy for a more intense workout. BCAA increases uptake of essential amino acid Tryptophan and reduce the synthesis and release of serotonin, which may delay fatigue during a longer or harder workout.

2. Build muscle

During a workout, muscles build and breakdown, and in time, fat breakdown to enable muscle tone build and fat loss, sculpturing the body.

The rate of muscle breakdown can be slowed during exercise with Leucine, an amino acid which stimulates protein synthesis and muscle tissue growth. So Leucine essentially primes the body preparing for muscle build and recover after a workout.

Taking BCAA can also increase the level of Dopamine seen with an increase of 2.5 times normal level of Phenylalanine. Dopamine is a reward neurotransmitter which make you feel motivated and satisfied when working out.

3. Assists with muscle soreness after exercise and prevents muscle damage

BCAA taken before exercise can reduce delayed onset muscle soreness (DOMS) as much as 20%. Intense exercise has the potential to damage muscle and is reflected in an increase in CK (creatinine kinase) and lactate dehydrogenase (LDH), indicators of muscle damage.

In a study by Coombes et al, the intake of BCAA's prior to a workout significantly decreased the post-exercise values of these enzymes, suggesting decreased muscle damage.

Neurotransmitter production

Amino acids are precursor molecules for both inhibitory and excitatory neurotransmitters. For example, Glutamate is the precursor for GABA; Histidine for histamine; Tyrosine for dopamine, noradrenaline and adrenalin; and Tryptophan for serotonin and melatonin.

Amino Acids are precursors of Neurotransmitters

Amino Acid	Neurotransmitters
Cysteine	Cysteic Acid
Glutamine	GABA, Glutamic Acid
Histidine	Histamine
Lysine	Pipecolic Acid
Phenylalanine	Phenylethylamine, Dopamine
Tyrosine	Dopamine, Noradrenaline, Adrenaline
Tryptophan	Serotonin, Melatonin

Like neurotransmitters, amino acids can possess inhibitory or excitatory characteristics.

Inhibitory Amino Acids	Excitatory Amino Acids
Alanine	Aspartic Acid
GABA	Glutamic Acid
Glycine	
Taurine	

Amino acids, such as Tryptophan, Phenylalanine, and Methionine, can influence pain threshold, mood, and sleep patterns. Tryptophan is the precursor of serotonin, which influences sleep patterns and mood.

Phenylalanine converts to the neurotransmitter Tyrosine and to the adrenal catecholamine, noradrenaline both of which influence mood and behavior.

Numerous studies suggest that Noradrenaline inhibits the release of adrenocorticotropic hormone (ACTH) by suppressing corticotropic releasing factor (CRF) secretion in the hypothalamus.[45]

Tyrosine supplementation assists in management of depression and HPA dysregulation.

The analgesic peptides, endorphins and enkephalins, are composed of amino acids; Methionine enkephalin has an analgesic potency 20 times that of morphine. Catecholamines must be methylated by S-adenosylmethionine (SAMe) for proper function; low levels of SAMe have been observed in some cases of depression.[46]

Glutamate is the principal excitatory neurotransmitter in the brain. Stimulation of synthesis of Glutamate has been implicated in chronic neurodegeneration and may be seen in disorders such as motor neurone disease (MND), amyotrophic lateral sclerosis (ALS) and Huntington's disease.[47]

Elevated levels of Tyrosine and Phenylalanine may contribute to the hallucinations in alcoholics and schizophrenics. Elevations in Tryptophan and Tyrosine have been correlated to efficacy of antidepressant therapy.

Brain regulation – The role of Glutamate

Glutamate is the principal excitatory neurotransmitter. It is associated with disorders such as amyotrophic lateral sclerosis (ALS) at Huntington's disease. Plasma Glutamate utilizes glutamic acid as an excitatory neurotransmitter.

Amino acids are degraded in the liver transforming glutamic acid to nitrogen and ammonia to produce urea via the urea cycle. Glutamine, therefore is involved in detoxification of ammonia which controls systemic pH regulation.

In acidic conditions, hydrolysis of Glutamine releases ammonia. Acidosis stimulates Glutamine uptake in the kidney which will in turn drive down plasma Glutamine.

High levels of plasma Glutamate are associated with headaches, inflammatory pain or infectious disease.

Interplay of Glutamate and Glutamine

Glutamate and Glutamine interact simultaneously in the citric acid cycle. Glutamine flux shifts between four principal processes:

1. gluconeogenesis
2. glutathione synthesis
3. Proline synthesis in the liver
4. Glutamine fructose six phosphate amino transferase (GFAT)

Glutamate is formed by transfer of amino groups from aspartate, Alanine and other amino acids by enzymes aspartate transaminase (AST) and Alanine transaminase (ALT).

Glutamic acid is produced when nitrogen or ammonia is transformed into urea. Glutamate carries nitrogen away from muscle tissue.

Glutamine is needed for detoxification of ammonia. During metabolic acidosis, Glutamine uptake is stimulated in the kidney leading to low plasma Glutamine.

As a result, low or high fasting plasma Glutamate and Glutamine may be found in chronic conditions such as headaches, fibromyalgia or infectious diseases.

Regulation of Glutamate

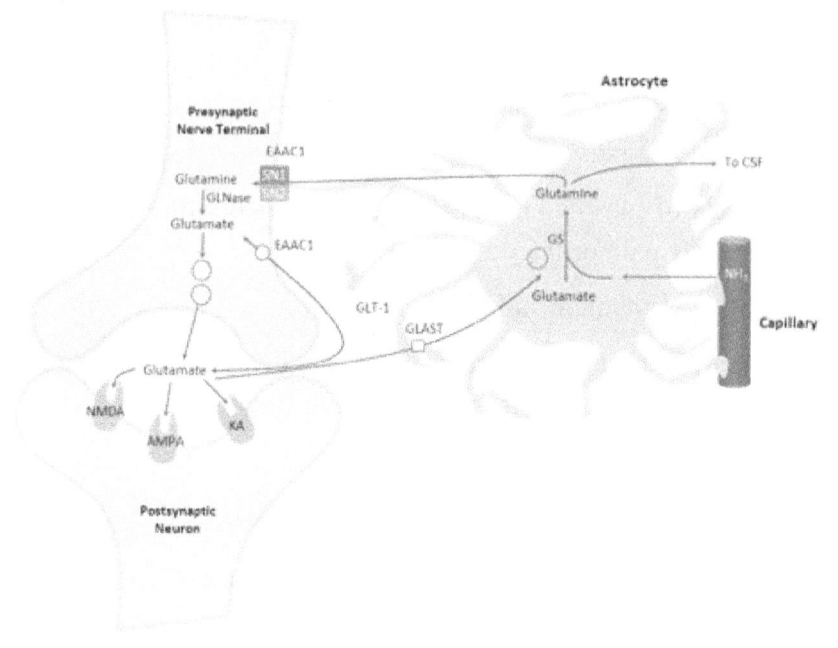

Glutamine, the most abundant amino acid in the body is released from the presynaptic neuron as Glutamate binding at one of 3 receptors, namely the N-methyl-D-aspartate (NMDA), AMPA, and kainite (KA) receptors.

Glutamate enhances neuroplasticity — the brain's capacity to change and grow — to learn, remember, and perform other cognitive functions.

Glutamate levels may be in excess due to:
- High levels of Glutamate accumulation in the brain.
- Glutamate receptors have become overly sensitive and thus are easily overstimulated

The brain has a remarkable ability to accumulate Glutamate, fortunately, however, safeguards are kept to regulate excess Glutamate from building up to dangerous levels in the brain.

NMDA activates Glutamate, D-Serine and Glycine. Synaptic Glutamate is taken up into neuronal astrocytes by Glutamate-aspartate transporter (GLAST). Blood ammonia stimulates the formation of Glutamine by Glutamine synthase. Transporters, SN 1 and SN2 are used to transfer Glutamine into presynaptic neurons which is then re-converted into Glutamate. Genetic mutations of SN1 and SN2 transporter systems simultaneously reduce elevation of plasma Glutamine, asparagine and Histidine. These patients may have difficulty maintaining normal tissue pH.

Glutamate blockers are used treat Glutamate toxicity. Pharmaceutical Glutamate blocking medication includes memantine and dextromethorphan.

Glutamate toxicity is associated with neurological disorders. Consumption of neurotoxic Glutamate agents can aggravate the nervous system.

Glutamine → Glutamate → GABA

Glutamate may reach neurotoxic levels due to:

- Glutamic acid decarboxylase (GAD) deficiency, the enzyme used to turn Glutamate into inhibitory GABA
- development of an autoimmune reaction to the GAD enzyme leading to poor conversion into GABA.
- Gluten intolerance, celiac disease, Hashimoto's disease, type 1 diabetes, and other autoimmune diseases are linked to GAD autoimmunity
- Co-factor deficiency, namely vitamin B6 (pyridoxine), an essential cofactor needed for conversion to GABA
- Genetic defect involved in Glutamate oversensitivity
- Traumatic stress can elevate Glutamate to abnormally high levels
- Intake of mood-altering substances disrupt the Glutamate-GABA balance
- Caffeine, the most widely used stimulant, increases Glutamate activity at the expense of GABA
- A brain injury or stroke causes Glutamate to flood the injured area[48]

Hormone production and release

Peptide research has grown to recognize the hormonal effects of amino acids. Tyrosine is an important precursor molecule for thyroid hormones. Arginine, Ornithine and Glutamine help stimulate the release of growth hormone.

A hormone called gluta-Taurine was discovered in the parathyroid gland of rats. Dr. L. Feuer and colleagues (1982, 1983) found that this peptide had highly selective actions on the thyroid and adrenal glands, organs involved in the response to stress.

Gluta-Taurine has Vit A-like effects antagonizing thyroid, adrenalin and adrenal hormones, more specifically, thyroxine and cortisone. Increased levels of Taurine have been found in hypothyroid patients.

Taurine also increased the effects of insulin. Use Taurine with caution in hypoglycemic patients.[49]

Kidney function and Nitrogen metabolism

The kidney plays a major role in amino acid metabolism and nutrition; amino acid reabsorption by renal tubules salvages about 70 g of filtered amino acids per day in a 70 kg man.

A measure of Creatinine in a urine sample can provide an excellent assessment of kidney function. High blood levels with low urine levels and a low 24-hour creatinine suggest subnormal renal clearance, while the opposite is seen in abnormally high renal clearance.

Nitrogen is a critical element for protein and DNA production, however excessive levels in the form of ammonia, are toxic to the body. Therefore, ensuring optimal levels of nitrogen in the body is essential to health.

Ornithine and Citrulline are two amino acids that are found in the urea cycle, a process which converts toxic ammonia to water-soluble urea.

In addition, Glutamine and Glutamate are involved in ammonia recycling in the body.

Whenever an amino acid is broken down, nitrogen is released, either as an amino group (-NH2) or as an ammonium ion (NH3+). Although nitrogen is essential to the body, an excess can form ammonia which is toxic to brain tissue. Resulting symptoms can include behavioral dysfunction, headaches, diarrhea, and CNS disturbances.

Ammonia is either transported to the liver where it is fixed as the nontoxic form urea in the urea cycle, or it is attached to the amino acid Glutamate, forming Glutamine. Glutamine can act as a nitrogen shuttle, removing nitrogen from the CNS.

Impaired ammonia detoxification may be indicated by elevated Glutamine, Asparagine, Alanine, or Glycine, as well as by elevated urea cycle intermediates (Arginine, Citrulline, Arginine-Succinate, Ornithine).[50]

Antioxidant protection

Glutathione is one of the most powerful antioxidants in the body. The Sulphur amino acids including Cysteine and Methionine are involved in its production. Deficiencies in these amino acids can result in oxidative stress.

Gastrointestinal Dysfunction

Amino acids analysis can indicate various aspects of gastrointestinal dysfunction.

Anserine and carnosine can result from deficient peptidase activity in the gut indicating incomplete digestive proteolysis. Altered intestinal permeability is commonly observed in these patients. Histidine is required to make histamine, the first digestive response in the stomach, low plasma or urine Histidine may also suggest maldigestion. Urine Hydroxyproline appears to be a hallmark for celiac disease.[51]

Gluconeogenesis

Glutamine tends to rise or fall with changes in demand for glucose production. When glucose elevation subsides, Glutamine is found to surpass or other amino acids including Alanine as a supplier for glucose synthesis.

Although plasma glucose is formed from Alanine all lactate release from skeletal muscle, only Glutamine contributes to a net gain of glucose.[52]

Detoxification

Phase II liver detoxification reactions ensure metabolites and toxins are water-soluble for excretion. In this process polar hydrophilic molecules are conjugated to the toxins.

The most common phase II reactions involve glutathione conjugation, amino acid conjugation (Taurine, Glycine), methylation, sulphation, acetylation and glucuronidation.

Amino acids either in a free or in peptide form needed for liver detoxification are Methionine, Cysteine, glutathione, Glutamine, Glycine, Alanine, Aspartic acid, and Taurine. These amino acids are involved in the body's detoxification of endogenous and exogenous compounds.

Deficiencies in any of these can result in impaired Phase II conjugation reactions, and accumulation of potentially toxic intermediates, and subsequent tissue damage and can manifest as neurological diseases, chemical intolerances, and chronic fatigue.[53]

Connective tissue and Collagen synthesis

Proline, Isoleucine, Leucine and Valine are required for connective tissue, muscle metabolism and tissue repair. Imbalances in these amino acids can lead to muscle atrophy, osteoporosis, poor wound healing and arthritis.

Collagen accounts for 25 to 30% of the body's protein. It is a major reservoir for Proline and hydroxy-Proline.

About half body's total Proline is contained in collagen. Nearly all protein contains Proline. Hydroxy-Proline plays a primary role in bone and connective tissue synthesis.

Proline may reduce the dietary requirements for Arginine, which is a lipid lowering amino acid. Arginine can be synthesized from Ornithine, and Ornithine from Proline. Vit C deficiency results in loss of Proline in the urine.[54]

Inflammation

Three amino acids are critical to antioxidant, anti-inflammatory functions are Cysteine, glutathione, and Taurine. Cysteine is considered to be the rate-limiting factor in the synthesis of the antioxidant tripeptide, Glutathione (GH).

GH is thought to be important during inflammatory response, influencing the production of phagocytes.

A study of reduced GH levels is associated with in a 30% decrease in these T cells. The decrease was prevented by treatment with N-acetylcysteine.

Decreased Cysteine has been reported in patients following severe trauma.

Taurine acts as a specific scavenger for the hypochlorite ion (OCl^-) during an inflammatory response. Taurine naturally limits the degree of inflammation and allows formation of stable chloro-amines from excess OCl^-.

When Taurine is low, the inflammatory response is enhanced and aldehydes may form, commonly resulting in aldehyde sensitivities and oxidative stress reactions.[55]

Cardiovascular Health

Impaired Methionine metabolism, particularly in homocystinuria has been found associated with coronary artery disease, peripheral and cerebral occlusive disease, myocardial infarction, and stroke. Homocysteine is an intermediate in the catabolism of Methionine, and it can either be remethylated into Methionine or broken down into Cysteine. When Methionine synthase enzyme in the SAMe methylation pathway does not function properly, Homocysteine can accumulate, which then contributes to oxidative damage and manifest as cardiovascular disease.[56]

Asymmetric Dimethyl-arginine (ADMA)

ADMA, an important marker of cardiovascular disease risk, is an endogenous inhibitor of angiogenesis. Arginine is the compound from which nitric oxide (NO) is formed and ADMA Is naturally occurring compound that inhibits NO synthases.

ADMA regulates nitric oxide production by modulating the availability for binding to nitric oxide synthase. Arginine is methylated to ADMA and is a precursor to Citrulline.

ADMA inhibits nitric oxide synthesis, and endothelial function contributing towards arteriosclerosis.

ADMA and Arginine are the two major regulators of nitric oxide synthesis and protection against cardiovascular disease. Arginine stimulates nitric oxide synthesis to overcome the inhibitory effects of ADMA. Low-fat meals tend to help the synthesis of ADMA. Antioxidants, vitamin B6, Vit B12, and folic acid help reduce ADMA.

Neuronal damage may increase the expression of ADMA to protect the neuronal cells from the effects of excess nitric oxide.[57]

The amino acid L-Arginine stimulates NO synthesis to overcome the inhibitory effects of high ADMA. Low fat meals help to reduce the synthesis of ADMA. Antioxidants, B-group vitamins and methylating cofactors enhance the removal of ADMA.

Cellular energy production

Many amino acids can be used as a fuel for energy when required. Glutamic acid, Aspartic acid, and Alanine form derivatives which are intermediate in the citric acid cycle.

Therefore, when imbalances of these different amino acids exist, energy production can be impaired, leading to fatigue, depression and muscle weakness.

Amino acids are required at each step of the Krebs cycle during digestion and assimilation and citric acid cycle in production of cellular energy as adenosine triphosphate, ATP.

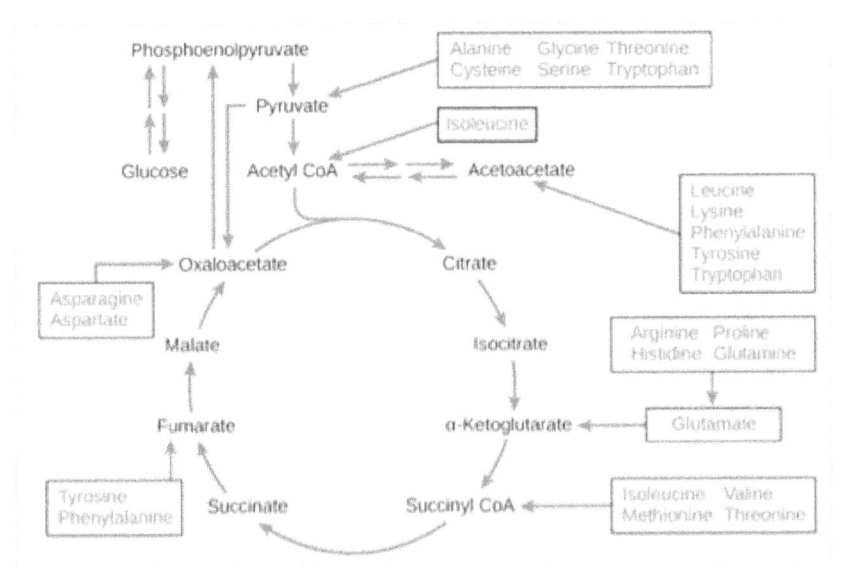

Image credit: "Connections of carbohydrate, protein, and lipid metabolic pathways," by OpenStax College, Biology, CC BY 4.0. Original work by Mikael Häggtröm

Amino Acids in General Medicine

The application of amino acid blends for health promotion is vital and effective.

Useful Amino Acid recipes for health conditions:

Disease	Amino acid
Acidosis	Carnitine
Addiction	Aspartic acid
Addictions – cigarette, cocaine	Tyrosine
Alcoholism	Glutamine
Alkalosis	Arginine, Lysine
ALS	Isoleucine, Leucine, mailing
Anemia	Carnitine, glutamic acid, histamine, Serine
Arrhythmia	Carnitine, Taurine
Arthritis	Histidine, Cysteine
Autism	Inositol
Bipolar disorder	choline, Inositol
BP	Arginine, carnitine, Taurine
Burns	Glutamine
Cardiovascular disease, angina	Arginine, carnitine, Creatine, Taurine
Cirrhosis	Arginine, carnitine, Glutamine, Taurine
Colitis	Carnitine, Glutamine
Cystic fibrosis	Arginine
Depression, aggression	Tryptophan, Aspartic acid, Glutamine, Inositol, Taurine, Arginine
Diabetes, hypoglycaemia	Arginine, carnitine, Inositol, Taurine, Alanine, GABA
Diabetic neuropathy	Inositol, carnitine
Epilepsy	Taurine, Tryptophan

Therapeutic Value of Amino Acids

Disease	Amino acid
Fatigue	Creatine, Isoleucine, Leucine, Valine
Gout	Glycine
Hair loss, alopecia	Cysteine, Arginine
Hangover	Alanine, Glutamine
Hangover	Alanine, Methionine
Herpes, cold sores	Lysine
Hyperlipidemia	carnitine, Lysine, Tryptophan, Taurine
Immune deficiency syndrome	Arginine, carnitine, Cysteine, Methionine
Impotence	Arginine
Insomnia	Tryptophan, Ornithine, searing, Glycine
Leg ulcer	Cysteine, Glycine, Threonine
Migraine	Tryptophan
Multiple Sclerosis	Choline, Threonine
Muscular dystrophy	Carnitine
Narcolepsy	Tyrosine
OCD	Tryptophan, Tyrosine, Phenylalanine
Phenylketonuria	Isoleucine, Leucine, Valine, Tryptophan, Tyrosine
Schizophrenia	Glycine, Isoleucine, Tryptophan, Methionine
Vitiligo	Phenylalanine
Wounds	Arginine, Aspartic acid

Diets high in Arginine and Glycine are associated with decreased cholesterol levels.

In Parkinson's disease, one would typically see high levels of Phosphatidylserine, Threonine, Methionine, Tyrosine, Sarcosine but lower levels of Threonine, Leucine and Tryptophan.

Testing of Amino Acids

An individual's amino acid status and requirements acids differ based on health conditions, dietary intake, exercise capacity, metabolic defects and genetics.

Amino acids and minerals form the basis of intracellular life. Most physiological pathways can be regulated, modulated and optimized using the core basics of life – amino acids and minerals. This is why I am so passionate about Amino Acids!

Tailoring an amino acid complex based on your own body chemistries personalizes amino acids for the individual. Amino acid analysis is the only way to establish the levels of amino acids in the body.

Why test amino acids?

Measurement of amino acid levels (serum or urine) can provide valuable information about the overall status of amino acid availability.

Recognizing biochemical individuality is a key factor in increasing chances for therapeutic success. Evaluation of amino acids allows for a treatment plan individualized for unique individual needs.

Patients who cannot sustain normal levels of amino acids in a fasting plasma may be candidates for individualized amino acid therapy.

Initial clinical use of amino acid testing was in neonatal inborn error detection such as phenylketonuria.

Amino acid testing is a powerful tool to not only determine underlying causes of disease, but to optimize health and slow down the aging process.

Test Amino Acid Status if you suspect:
- Protein and nutrient cofactor adequacy
- Enzyme functionality
- Predisposition to various degenerative disorders
- Wasting syndromes
- Gastro-intestinal dysfunction
- Neurological disorders
- Impairments in detoxification
- Inborn errors of metabolism

Which Amino Acid test is best?

Testing amino acid levels in both plasma and urine would provide the most comprehensive assessment of amino acid metabolism in patients. Results would highlight both impairment of amino acid production and excretion. Urine testing is the preferred specimen type due to ease of collection.

Plasma versus urine testing versus blood Spot

The **urinary** amino acid test, in contrast to plasma testing, provides reading of the total daily levels of amino acids rather than just a measure at one moment in time. Urinary testing is not affected by circadian rhythms. Another advantage of urinary amino acid testing is that it is more sensitive and therefore can detect marginal imbalances.

When detecting metabolic disorders due to genetic polymorphisms, micronutrient deficiencies or toxic abnormalities, urine amino acid testing is preferred.

24-hour urine amino acid analysis reveals amino acid metabolism throughout a 24-hour period. Valuable for evaluating amino acids that reveal tissue degradation. Urine amino acid analysis reveals metabolism of amino acids due to daily activity.

Hydroxy Lysine and hydroxyproline are released from collagen of connective tissue and bone. Urine analysis is the preferred specimen for detecting abnormalities of some non-essential amino acids.

Plasma testing should be considered in patients with poor renal function, any known kidney disease and in any situation in which the 24-hour urinary collection is impractical. Plasma testing will reflect the state of dynamic flux of amino acids leaving skeletal muscle and entering sites of utilization in the liver, brain or other tissues.

Plasma assessments of amino acids are the preferred specimen for essential amino acids insufficiency. **Taurine** is the only notable **exception** being higher in blood due to a high concentration in erythrocytes. Some amino acids such as Hydroxylysine and Hydroxyproline are released from breakdown of collagen and bone. Urinary testing may be challenging to determine deficiency states in comparison to a blood sample.

Urine testing is preferable for assessment of non-essential amino acids. In addition, correction of concentration gradients with a creatinine measure based on volume variation of urine is prone to error in the young, immune-compromised and palliative care patients.

Fasting blood plasma has the greatest validation of scientific studies. It provides higher levels of reliability that shift individual amino acid demands.

Blood Spot testing is recommended for essential and conditionally essential amino acids.

Levels of amino acids tested in blood spot, plasma or blood are comparable.

Collection of samples for testing

It is important to follow collection instructions as stipulated in the kit provided.

Urine testing

Discontinue all non-essential medications, amino acid supplements, protein powders and any products containing the artificial sweetener aspartame four days prior to specimen collection. Do not collect urine during menstruation. Do not collect urine if you have a urinary tract infection. Wait until it is resolved. Decrease fluid intake to avoid excessive dilution of the urine (for eg. < 2 Litres). Do not perform this test if you have a kidney disorder or are on diuretics. Your healthcare provider will tell you whether or not to discontinue any drug or activities that may interfere with the test.

Plasma testing

Fasting blood sample is not required. However, to avoid false negative reading following a protein rich or protein variable diet, consider a fasting blood collection.

Analytes measured in various samples

Plasma/Blood Amino Acids analytes measured:

1-methylHistidine, 3-methylHistidine, Alanine, alpha-aminoadipate, alpha-amino-N-butyrate, ammonia, Anserine, Arginine, arginosuccinate, asparagine, aspartate, beta-Alanine, beta-aminoisobutyrate, carnosine, Citrulline, cystathionine, cystine, ethanolamine, gaba, Glutamate, Glutamine, Glycine, Histidine, Homocysteine, hydroxyProline, Isoleucine, Leucine, Lysine, Methionine, Ornithine, Phenylalanine, phosphoethanolamine, Phosphoserine, Proline, sarcosine, Serine, Taurine, Threonine, Tryptophan, Tyrosine, urea, Valine, Glutamine/Glutamate.

Blood Spot Essential & Non Essential Amino Acids analytes measured: Arginine, Asparagine, Aspartic Acid, Citrulline, Glutamate, Glutamine, Glycine, Histidine, Isoleucine, Leucine, Lysine, Methionine, Ornithine, Phenylalanine, Serine, Taurine, Threonine, Tryptophan, Tyrosine, Valine

Blood Spot Essential Amino Acids analytes measured: **Arginine, Histidine, Isoleucine, Leucine, Lysine, Methionine, Phenylalanine, Taurine, Threonine, Tryptophan, Valine**

Urine (spot or 24 hour urine) Amino Acids analytes measured: 1-methylHistidine, 3-methylHistidine, Alanine, Alpha-Aminoadipate, Alpha-Amino-N-Butyrate, Ammonia, Anserine, Arginine, Arginosuccinate, Asparagine, Aspartate, Beta-Alanine, Beta-Aminoisobutyrate, Carnosine, Citrulline, Cystathionine, Cysteine, Cystine, Ethanolamine, Gaba, Glutamate, Glutamine, Glycine, Histidine, Homocysteine, HydroxyProline, Isoleucine, Leucine, Lysine, Methionine, Ornithine, Phenylalanine, Phospho-ethanolamine, Phosphoserine, Proline, Sarcosine, Serine, Taurine, Threonine, Tryptophan, Tyrosine, Urea, Valine, Glutamine/Glutamate.

Testing Preference for amino acid testing

Some amino acids such as Hydroxylysine and Hydroxyproline are released from breakdown of collagen and bone. Urinary testing may be challenging to determine deficiency states in comparison to a blood sample. Urine testing is preferable for assessment of non-essential amino acids. In addition, correction of concentration gradients with a creatinine measure based on volume variation of urine is prone to error in the young, immune-compromised and palliative care patients. Taurine is the only notable exception being higher in blood due to a high concentration in erythrocytes. Testing of amino acids were and still are used to detect neonatal inborn errors such as phenylketonuria.

Preference of specimens for Amino Acid Testing:[58]

Function	Amino acids	specimen
Essential amino acids	Leucine, Isoleucine, Valine, Phenylalanine, Lysine, Threonine, Methionine, Tryptophan	plasma, blood spot
Conditionally essential amino acids	Arginine, Tyrosine, Histidine, Glycine, Serine	plasma, blood spot
Neurologic markers	Tryptophan, Methionine, GABA, Tyrosine, Phenylalanine	plasma, blood spot
Cardiovascular	Taurine	plasma
Nutrient and vitamin markers	Histadine, Phenylalanine, Anserine, Carnosine	plasma. blood spot, urine
Bone loss, collagen markers	HydroxyProline, Hydroxylysine, Cysteine, 3-Methyl Histadine	urine
Gut Dysbiosis markers	B-Alanine	urine

Amino acid transport

Plasma proteins are responsible for transporting hormones, minerals and vital elements from the blood to the tissues. Just as iron is transported by transferrin, hormones by sex hormone binding globulin, copper by ceruloplasmin, amino acids levels are also influenced by transporters.

Amino acid transporters reside in plasma membranes and typically exchange sodium irons (active transport) and/or amino acids (passive transport). The transporters are classified as system A or system N (SN) and the S class is further differentiated into SN1 and SN2.

The transporters are coded by single genes or a number of separate genes which can be up- or down- regulated which respond to external signals which influence amino acid utilization such as nitric oxide or insulin. Polymorphisms in SN1 and SN2 transporter proteins can be the origin of abnormalities in plasma Glutamine.

The physiological substrates for SN1 and SN2 amino acid transporters are Glycine, asparagine and histamine. Whereas SN2 transporter is Serine, Alanine and Glycine. Individuals with such patterns have difficulty in maintaining normal tissue pH.

Cofactors for Amino acids

Cofactor requirements are essential for therapeutic function of amino acids. Vit B6 and iron for example, is needed to manufacture serotonin from Tryptophan.

A synergistic blend of amino acids may form part of physiological benefit. For example, branched chain amino acids, Valine, Leucine and Isoleucine are released from skeletal muscle during strenuous exercise. Supplementation of BCAA's is therefore recommended during exercise.

Basic amino acids such as histamine, Lysine, Arginine are abundant in histones and bind to negatively charged DNA when amino acids are degraded in the liver.

Large neutral amino acids like Tryptophan, Tyrosine, Phenylalanine, Leucine, Isoleucine and Methionine compete for intestinal absorption and transport at the blood brain barrier.

When amino acids are degraded in the liver, glutamic acid is produced and ammonia is transformed into urine via the urea cycle. Glutamate carries nitrogen away from exercising muscle via alpha ketoglutarate. Glutamine is involved in detoxification of ammonia. Glutamine and Glycine regulate systemic pH in the kidney, liver and brain during food intake.

Digestion of Protein

Ingested protein is digested to release amino acids which are absorbed into the bloodstream in the small intestine. The efficiency of protein digestions depends on adequate hydrochloric acid to initiate poached protein denaturation and stimulate pancreatic and biliary fluid flow. Abnormally low or high amino acid levels can be caused by dietary deficiencies of protein and micronutrients. Variations in metabolic demands by hormones or toxic factors that increase the loss.

Interpretation of Amino Acid Analysis

What does it mean to have a low or high level of an amino acid?

How are amino acids synthesized or managed?

Where in the diet can an amino acid be found?

In this chapter, you will view interpretation of amino acids with its correlation to diet choices and disease states. These charts are available as easy to use printable PDF formats.

Alchemy of Amino Acids

Amino Acid	Properties	Biosynthesis	Low	Treatment	High	Treatment	Food Sources
1-MethylHistidine *Amino Acid Metabolite*	The enzyme, carnosinase, splits Anserine into b-Alanine and 1-M-hitadine serve as an objective indicator of meat ingestion	Derived from Anserine	Increased oxidative effects in skeletal muscle Zinc is required for the normal conversion to B-Alanine plus 1-methylhistidine		Meat and poultry consumption Low methyltransferase enzyme activity leading to low Histidine levels Vitamin B12 and folate are catalysts for the methyltransferase enzymes. Inadequate methyl group transfer leads to low Histidine levels, impaired Methionine metabolism. inhibit carnosinase	Vit E Vit B12 Me-Folate Vit E DMG Zinc	Meat
3-MethylHistidine *Amino Acid Metabolite*	Serve as a marker of muscle degradation reflects dietary meat intake	3-methylhistidine (3-MH) is formed by methylation of Histidine	Dystrophic muscles	BCAA's	Active catabolism of muscle protein Low antioxidant status Folic acid deficiency	Vit E Vit B12 Me-Folate Vit E DMG Zinc	Meat
Alanine *Non-essential amino acid*	Glucose metabolism nitrogen metabolism Enhances the immune system. Phase II liver detoxification	Transamination from pyruvic acid and glutamic acid in the liver	Adrenal fatigue Anorexia Calorie restriction Diabetes (due to its role in gluconeogenesis) Hepatitis Hypoglycemia Muscle loss	Increase dietary protein Alanine branched chain amino acids Leucine, Isoleucine and Valine	Chronic Fatigue Syndrome - inadequate cellular energy substrates renal sclerosis osteoporosis Adrenal stress Manganese deficiency (if alpha-aminoadipic acid, Isoleucine, Leucine, Tyrosine, or Valine are also elevated) Vitamin B6 deficiency (if Alanine, Aspartic acid, Glycine, Isoleucine, Leucine, Ornithine, Serine, Threonine, Tyrosine or Valine are also elevated) Hypoglycemia or exercise muscle wasting branched-chain amino acids.	Vitamin B6 Manganese branched-chain amino acids Investigate glucose and insulin levels Vitamin B6	Meat, Poultry, Fish, Egg, Dairy products, Avocado

Interpretation of Amino Acid Analysis

Amino Acid	Properties	Biosynthesis	Low	Treatment	High	Treatment	Food Sources
Alpha-Aminoadipic Acid *Amino Acid Metabolite*			Predictor of the development of diabetes	Lysine	Impaired Lysine metabolism Intestinal dysbiosis (if beta-Alanine, GABA or ethanolamine are also elevated) Manganese deficiency (if Isoleucine, Leucine, Tyrosine, or Valine are also elevated) Vitamin B6 deficiency (if Alanine, beta-Alanine, Aspartic acid, beta-aminoisobutyric acid, cystathione, Glycine, homocystine, Isoleucine, Leucine, Ornithine, Serine, Threonine, Tyrosine or Valine are also elevated).	Manganese α-Ketoglutaric acid Vitamin B6 Probiotics Investigate & treat intestinal dysbiosis	
Alpha-Amino-N-Butyric Acid *Amino Acid Metabolite*		Derived from Threonine	Threonine deficiency Cofactor insufficiencies	α-Ketoglutaric acid Vitamin B6	under-conversion of alpha-amino-N-butyric acid to succinyl CoA for use in the citric acid cycle Cofactor deficiencies	Biotin Vitamin B12	
Ammonia	Compound of nitrogen and hydrogen		Check kidney function		Intestinal dysbiosis (if alpha-aminoadipic acid, beta-Alanine, GABA or ethanolamine are also elevated) Protein overload (if urea is also elevated) Specimen decay (if normal urea).		

Alchemy of Amino Acids

Amino Acid	Properties	Biosynthesis	Low	Treatment	High	Treatment	Food Sources
Anserine *Amino Acid Metabolite*					High dietary poultry intake. Maldigestion or leaky gut (if carnosine is high & if low or low normal essential amino acids). Bone and connective tissue disorders (if carnosine, hydroxylysine and hydroxyproline are also elevated). Zinc deficiency	Investigate maldigestion & leaky gut. Zinc (15mg/day). Zn, 30 mg	
Arginine *Semi-essential amino acid*	Enhances the immune system. May lower cholesterol support the cardiovascular system insulin and growth hormone release. Neutralizes ammonia in the liver. Used in the synthesis of GABA and Creatine major component of collagen. Manganese activates an arginase enzyme		Angina Arthritis Constipation Diabetes or insulin dysregulation Erectile dysfunction Fatigue Fatty liver Hair loss High blood pressure Low libido Low growth hormone Low muscle mass Migraines Poor wound healing Skin rash hyperammonemia (correlate with citric acid and orotic acid in urine) Adrenal stress (if Tryptophan & Tyrosine are also low)	Arginine	block in the urea cycle (if urea is low, Glutamine is high and Arginine, Citrulline, or Ornithine is also elevated; Manganese deficiency (if Arginine is elevated in comparison to Ornithine) Functional block in urea cycle (deficiency of arginase) Liver / kidney failure	Reduce protein intake Manganese	Poultry, meats, fish, beans, (esp. Soy), grains, nuts & seeds, gelatin, cereals (esp. Buckwheat groats, oatmeal and millet), milk, cheese and egg, wheat germ, some vegetables (esp. Green peas, asparagus, broccoli, swiss chard, corn, white potato, onion and spinach), avocado, chocolate

Interpretation of Amino Acid Analysis

Amino Acid	Properties	Biosynthesis	Low	Treatment	High	Treatment	Food Sources
Argininosuccinic acid					Impaired ammonia detoxification (if urea is low and any of the following amino acids are elevated: Arginine, Citrulline or Ornithine)		
Asparagine *Non-essential amino acid*		Closely related to Aspartic acid (is the amide form)	functional magnesium deficiency, as magnesium is required for the conversion of Aspartic acid to asparagine Decreased growth Decreased muscle mass	Magnesium	Problems with purine and therefore protein synthesis.		Asparagus, dairy products, beef, poultry, egg, fish, beans, nuts, seeds, soy and whole grains
Aspartic Acid (Aspartate) *Non-essential amino acid*	Plays an important role in the citric acid cycle and in ATP production Utilized in phase II liver detoxification excitatory neurotransmitter Involved in the urea cycle. Can be converted to oxaloacetate using B6 and a-KG and thus enter the Krebs cycle	Produced from Glutamate by the vitamin B6 dependent enzyme serum glutamic oxaloacetic transaminase (SGOT)	Depression Maldigestion Fatigue - Decreased cellular energy generation Impaired phase II liver detoxification inhibits ammonia detoxification in the urea cycle	alpha-ketoglutaric acid Vit B6	May be associated with Epilepsy and Stroke	Magnesium Zinc	Milk and dairy products, especially cheese Egg, meat (chicken, pork, beef, etc) Fish (salmon, halibut, sardines, mackerel, etc.) Nuts (walnuts, pistachios, almonds, chestnuts) Cereals (oats, corn) Sprouting seeds.

Alchemy of Amino Acids

Amino Acid	Properties	Biosynthesis	Low	Treatment	High	Treatment	Food Sources
Beta-Alanine *Amino Acid Metabolite*	Utilized in phase II liver detoxification		Tingling, skin crawling, burning lips/ears/nose sensation	Beta-alanine	possible bowel toxicity due to β-Alanine production by intestinal bacteria and/or Candida albicans Impaired phase II liver detoxification (especially if Methionine, cystathionine & Taurine levels are abnormal) Intestinal dysbiosis (if alpha-aminoadipic acid, GABA or ethanolamine are also elevated) Vitamin B6 deficiency (if Alanine, alpha-aminoadipic acid, Aspartic acid, beta-aminoisobutyric acid, cystathione, Glycine, homocystine, Isoleucine, Leucine, Ornithine, Serine, Threonine, Tyrosine or Valine are also elevated).	Vitamin B6 - facilitate amine group transfer Lactobacillus acidolphilus and Bifidobacteria Investigate & treat intestinal dysbiosis	
Beta-Aminoisobutyric Acid *Amino Acid Metabolite*	Excitatory neurotransmitter				Vitamin B6 deficiency (if Alanine, alpha-aminoadipic acid, beta-Alanine, Aspartic acid, cystathione, Glycine, homocystine, Isoleucine, Leucine, Ornithine, Serine, Threonine, Tyrosine or Valine are also elevated) Vitamin B12 deficiency (if beta-Alanine, Glycine or homocystine are also elevated)	Vit B6 Vit B12	

Interpretation of Amino Acid Analysis

Amino Acid	Properties	Biosynthesis	Low	Treatment	High	Treatment	Food Sources
Carnosine *Amino Acid Metabolite*	Involved in the urea cycle concentrated in muscle and brain tissue	Dipeptide of the amino acids beta-Alanine and Histidine			Neurological development problems. Sensory polyneuropathy. Maldigestion or leaky gut (if Anserine is high & if low or normal essential amino acids). Bone and connective tissue disorders (if Anserine, hydroxylysine and hydroxyproline are also elevated). Carnosinase enzyme deficiency. Zinc deficiency. Inherited carnosinase enzyme deficits lead to neurological development problems and sensory polyneuropathy	Investigate maldigestion & leaky gut Zinc	
Creatine *Nitrogenous organic compound*	Recycling of ATP ph buffer increase maximum power and performance	Produced from Arginine and Glycine	May be observed in people with small muscle mass Low meat diets		Strenuous exercise kidney problems		

121

Alchemy of Amino Acids

Amino Acid	Properties	Biosynthesis	Low	Treatment	High	Treatment	Food Sources
Cystathionine *Sulphur Amino Acid*		Produced by the transsulphur-ion pathway which converts Homocyste-ine into cystathionine	Coronary artery disease (if homocystine is also elevated and Methionine, Cysteine or Taurine are abnormal) Connective and bone tissue disorders (if homocystine is also elevated)		Neurological & behavioural disorders Vitamin B6 deficiency (if Alanine, alpha-aminoadipic acid, beta-Alanine, Aspartic acid, beta-aminoisobutyric acid, Glycine, homocystine, Isoleucine, Leucine, Ornithine, Serine, Threonine, Tyrosine or Valine are also elevated) Folic acid deficiency (if 1-methylHistidine, 3-methylHistidine, cystathionine, Glycine, Histidine, homocystine, Methionine, sarcosine, or Serine are also elevated)	Vit B6 Me-Folate	
Citrulline	An intermediate in the urea cycle Essential for detoxifying and removing ammonia from muscle and liver cells.	Made from Ornithine and carbamoyl phosphate in one of the central reactions in the urea cycle			Magnesium deficiency, as magnesium is required to convert Citrulline into argininosuccinic acid block in the urea cycle (if Glutamine is high, urea is low and any of the following amino acids are elevated: Arginine, Citrulline or Ornithine).can indicate a functional enzyme block in the urea cycle, leading to an ammonia buildup.	Magnesium Aspartic Acid Low protein diet	

Interpretation of Amino Acid Analysis

Amino Acid	Properties	Biosynthesis	Low	Treatment	High	Treatment	Food Sources
Cysteine and Cystine *sulphur containing semi-essential amino acid*	Required for the formation of coenzyme A, insulin, heparin and biotin production of important antioxidants and detoxifying molecules e.g. Metallothionein, glutathione phase II liver detoxification	Synthesized from methionine. Cystine consists of two Cysteine molecules joined together	AIDS. Cardiovascular disease. Pulmonary disease. May impair Taurine synthesis dietary deficiency of Methionine and/or Cysteine. Chronic exposure to sulfhydryl reactive metals (eg. mercury, cadmium, arsenic) or toxic chemicals. Oxidative stress or insufficient antioxidants (vitamins E and C) (especially if cystine is elevated compared to Cysteine). Inflammation. Impaired Methionine metabolism (inadequate folic acid, vitamin B12, vitamin B6, magnesium) possible dietary deficiency of Methionine and/or cystine. Low cystine can impair Taurine synthesis.	N-Acetyl Cysteine (except in cystinuria, intestinal candidiasis or insulin-dependent diabetes	Cardiovascular disease. Excessive dietary cystine intake. Impaired Cysteine metabolism (cystine is converted to Cysteine by a vitamin B2 and copper-dependent enzyme). Oxidative stress or insufficient antioxidants if cystine is elevated compared to Cysteine. Impaired phase II liver detoxification (especially if Methionine, cystathionine & Taurine levels are abnormal). Vitamin B6 is required for production of Taurine from Cysteine excessive dietary intake or impaired cystine metabolism. Converted to Cysteine (reduced cystine) via a B2 and copper-dependent step. Cystine is a major component of tissue antioxidant mechanisms.	Vitamin B2 Antioxidants Liver detoxification Check Homocysteine levels	Meat, poultry, fish, grains, beans (esp. Soy), egg, nuts & seeds, milk, cheese, cereals (esp. Couscous)

123

Alchemy of Amino Acids

Amino Acid	Properties	Biosynthesis	Low	Treatment	High	Treatment	Food Sources
Gamma-aminobutyric acid (GABA) *Non-essential amino acid*	Inhibitory neurotransmitter	Formed from glutamic acid GABA is metabolized to form succinic acid, which is a Kreb's cycle intermediate	Attention-deficit hyperactivity disorder (ADHD) Epilepsy Hypertension Panic attacks Premenstrual Syndrome	GABA Glutamine Glycine Fat soluble vitamins	decreased ability to convert GABA to succinic acid (a Krebs cycle intermediate) Intestinal dysbiosis (if alpha-aminoadipic acid, beta-Alanine, or ethanolamine are also elevated)	α-Ketoglutaric acid Vitamin B6.	
Glutamic Acid (Glutamate) *Non-essential amino acid*	Excitatory neurotransmitter Important for nitrogen homeostasis metabolism of sugars and fats component of folic acid	Synthesized from a number of amino acids including Ornithine and Arginine When aminated, glutamic acid forms Glutamine precursor of glutathione	Alcoholism Epilepsy Fatigue Mental retardation Muscular dystrophy Renal wasting Schizophrenia Mild hyperammonemia (especially if high Glutamine). Low protein, high complex carbohydrate diet	If ammonia toxicity is confirmed, low protein, high complex carbohydrate diet is suggested. vitamin B6 α-ketoglutarate branch chain amino acids	Headaches Neurological disorders. Possible under-conversion to α-ketoglutarate in liver for use in citric acid cycle Excessive intake of dietary protein Vitamin B6 insufficiency or impaired metabolism of vitamin B6 Renal transport defect (if Aspartic acid and α-aminoadipic acid are also elevated). Under-conversion to alpha-ketoglutarate for Krebs cycle	Niacin (Vitamin B3) Vitamin B6	Foods matured, cured, or preserved, such as matured cheeses Fish sauce Soy sauce and soy protein Mushrooms Ripe tomatoes Broccoli Peas Walnuts

124

Interpretation of Amino Acid Analysis

Amino Acid	Properties	Biosynthesis	Low	Treatment	High	Treatment	Food Sources
Glutamine *Nonessential amino acid*	Most abundant amino acid in the body. The formation of Glutamine from Glutamate protects against excess accumulation of cytotoxic ammonia in the brain build and maintain the muscles fuel source for cells lining the intestines immune function stimulate growth hormone	Glutamine is derived from Histidine Derived directly from dietary protein Formed endogenously by addition of ammonia to Glutamate	Protein-deficient diet Chronic alcoholism Impaired phase II liver detoxification Maldigestion Fasting Fatigue GI inflammation Malabsorption Strict dieting Ulcers Negative nitrogen balance Renal acidosis; associated with increased renal glutaminase activity and increased ammonia excretion Cirrhosis, and weight loss associated with AIDS and cancer	Increase dietary protein Ensure optimal digestion and absorption (e.g. HCl, Digestive Enzymes) Glutamine	Vitamin B6 deficiency Ammonia accumulation (if low or low normal glutamic acid) Impaired ammonia detoxification (if urea is low and any of the following amino acids are elevated: Arginine, Citrulline or Ornithine). Ammonia accumulation suspected, if low or low normal glutamic acid marker of vitamin B6 deficiency Extra a-KG needed to combine with ammonia and to make up for energy deficit caused by overutilization of a-KG to deal with toxic ammonia levels	If ammonia toxicity is confirmed, low protein, high complex carbohydrate diet is suggested vitamin B6 α-ketoglutarate	Raw parsley, cabbage and spinach. Beef, poultry, pork, fish and organ meats, Milk, yogurt, ricotta cheese and cottage cheese, goats milk, beans

Amino Acid	Properties	Biosynthesis	Low	Treatment	High	Treatment	Food Sources
Glutamine: Glutamate Ratio *for urinary sample only*			Specimen decay When aged, warmed or improperly preserved, urine Glutamine readily breaks down to Glutamate and ammonia, hence the test results may not be truly representative for this patient high levels of Glutamate can be associated with gout or metabolic acidosis Chronic alcoholism negative nitrogen balance	Treat with High Glutamate protocol			

Interpretation of Amino Acid Analysis

Amino Acid	Properties	Biosynthesis	Low	Treatment	High	Treatment	Food Sources
Glycine *Non-essential amino acid*	Inhibitory neurotransmitter. Supports glycogen storage. Promotes tissue repair. Involved in nucleic acid (DNA, RNA) formation. Utilised in phase II liver detoxification. Glycine is part of the nitrogen pool and important in gluconeogenesis	Manufactured from Serine and Threonine	Fat maldigestion especially if low or high Taurine. Impaired phase II liver detoxification if low Glycine, Glutamine or Aspartic acid. Generalized tissue loss. Decreased growth, muscle mass. Fat maldigestion especially if low or high Taurine. Epilepsy. Hyperactivity. Manic depression. Muscle atrophy. Prostatic hypertrophy	Glycine. Fat soluble vitamins	Increased risk of kidney stones (oxalic acid). Decreased metabolism of Glycine for pyruvate or gluconeogenesis production or gluconeogenesis. Fat maldigestion (if elevated in the urinary sample only). Vitamin B6 deficiency (if Alanine, alpha-aminoadipic acid, beta-Alanine, Aspartic acid, beta-aminoisobutyric acid, cystathione, homocystine, Isoleucine, Leucine, Ornithine, Serine, Threonine, Tyrosine or Valine are also elevated). Folic acid deficiency (if 1-methylHistidine, 3-methylHistidine, cystathionine, Glycine, Histidine, homocysteine, Methionine, sarcosine, or Serine are also elevated)	Folic acid. Vitamin B6. Vitamin B2 - efficient metabolism of Glycine to pyruvic acid for oxidation and for glutathione synthesis or gluconeogenesis. Vitamin B5. Fat soluble vitamins	Fish. Meat. Beans. Dairy products.

Alchemy of Amino Acids

Amino Acid	Properties	Biosynthesis	Low	Treatment	High	Treatment	Food Sources
Histidine *semi-essential amino acid*	Stimulates the production gastric acid. Needed for blood cells and hemoglobin. Essential for tissue growth and repair. Important for myelin sheath maintenance	Precursor for histamine & carnosine	Protein-deficient diet. Hypochlorhydria from deficient histamine. May lead to iron and manganese deficiency. Maldigestion. Folate deficiency. Poor dietary intake. Malabsorption. Rheumatoid arthritis. Impaired ability of protein digestion. Salicylate and steroids may lower Histidine	Digestive support (e.g. HCl, Digestive enzymes. Investigate and treat mineral deficiencies (e.g. Folic acid, Manganese, Iron). Histidine. Folate	Excessive protein intake. Folic acid deficiency (if 1-methylHistidine, 3-methylHistidine, cystathionine, Glycine, Histidine, Homocysteine, Methionine, sarcosine, or Serine are also elevated). Excessive protein intake. Muscle protein breakdown (correlate with high 3-methyl-Histidine)	Reduce protein intake.	Meats, poultry, fish, beans (esp. Soy), cheese, milk, egg, grains, nuts & seeds, cereals, white potato
Hydroxylysine	Most widely known component of collagen. A marker of bone and connective tissue resorption crucial role in stabilizing collagen and connective tissue structure	Biosynthesized from Lysine via oxidation by lysyl hydroxylase enzymes			Collagen breakdown. Connective and bone tissue disorders. Vitamin C deficiency. See hydroxyProline results indicative of connective and bone tissue breakdown. Arthritis. Blood vessel damage. Bruising. Osteoporosis. Wrinkles	Chondroitin sulphate. Manganese. Vitamin C. Iron manganese	

Interpretation of Amino Acid Analysis

Amino Acid	Properties	Biosynthesis	Low	Treatment	High	Treatment	Food Sources
Hydroxyproline	A marker of bone and connective tissue resorption crucial role in stabilizing collagen and connective tissue structure				Collagen breakdown Connective and bone tissue disorders Vitamin C deficiency See hydroxylysine results - another indicator bone resorption via collagen breakdown Arthritis Blood vessel damage Bruising Osteoporosis Wrinkles	Chondroitin sulphate Manganese Vitamin C Iron manganese	

Alchemy of Amino Acids

Amino Acid	Properties	Biosynthesis	Low	Treatment	High	Treatment	Food Sources
Isoleucine *essential amino acid branched-chain structural amino acid that like Leucine and Valine*	Regulates blood sugar and energy levels Required for hemoglobin formation Aids in increasing growth hormone production		Zinc deficiency Maldigestion or leaky gut (if low (or low normal) essential amino acids) Bone and connective tissue disorders (if Leucine or Valine are also low, and hydroxylysine and hydroxyproline are elevated). hypoglycemia Muscle atrophy - loss of muscle mass or inability to build muscle	Zinc Digestive support (e.g. HCl, Digestive enzymes)	Excessive consumption of amino acids Incomplete metabolism of amino acids Vitamin B6 deficiency (if Alanine, Aspartic acid, Glycine, Leucine, Ornithine, Serine, Threonine, Tyrosine or Valine are also elevated) Manganese deficiency (if Alanine, Leucine, Tyrosine or Valine are also elevated). large intake of this AA or incomplete metabolism of it. If other BCAAs are high, add vitamin B6 to aid metabolism.	Vitamin B6 Manganese Check for insulin resistance.	Poultry, meats, fish, beans (esp. Soy), milk, cheese, egg, grains, cereals (esp. Millet), nuts & seeds, some vegetables (esp. Swiss chard, corn, green peas, white potato and spinach), avocado, spinach

Interpretation of Amino Acid Analysis

Amino Acid	Properties	Biosynthesis	Low	Treatment	High	Treatment	Food Sources
Leucine *essential amino acid branched-chain structural amino acid like Isoleucine and Valine*	Aids in tissue repair. Aids in increasing growth hormone production. Regulates blood sugar and energy levels		Associated Symptoms and Conditions: Hypoglycemia. Muscle atrophy. Catabolism of skeletal muscle. Maldigestion or leaky gut. Bone and connective tissue disorders (if Leucine or Valine are also low, and hydroxylysine and hydroxyproline are elevated). Catabolism of skeletal muscle seen as loss of muscle mass (e.g. stress, critical illness). High alcohol intake potential catabolism of skeletal muscle. Check 3-methyl-Histidine to confirm this.	Treatment Considerations: A balanced or custom mixture of essential amino acids. Zinc supplementation (15mg/day). Digestive support (e.g. HCl, Digestive enzymes, L-Glutamine, Probiotics).	large intake of this AA or incomplete metabolism of it. If other BCAAs are high, add vitamin B6 to aid metabolism. May Indicate: Excessive consumption of amino acids. Incomplete metabolism of amino acids. Vitamin B6 deficiency (if Alanine, alpha-aminoadipic acid, beta-Alanine, Aspartic acid, beta-aminoisobutyric acid, cystathione, Glycine, Homocysteine, Isoleucine, Ornithine, Serine, Threonine, Tyrosine or Valine are also elevated). Manganese deficiency (if Alanine, alpha-aminoadipic acid, Isoleucine, Tyrosine, or Valine are also elevated). Excessive dietary intake of BCAAs; Inadequate vitamin B6, required for metabolism	Treatment Considerations: Vitamin B6 100mg/day. Manganese 15mg/day. Check for insulin resistance. B6, 100 mg; Check for insulin insensitivity	Chicken. Fish. Asparagus., cheese, egg, grains, cereals (esp. Millet), nuts seeds, gelatin, some vegetables (esp. Sweet potato, white potato, spinach, corn, green peas, asparagus, broccoli, swiss chard, mushrooms and tomato), avocado, wheat germ.

Amino Acid	Properties	Biosynthesis	Low	Treatment	High	Treatment	Food Sources
Lysine *glucogenic essential amino acid*	Involved in the synthesis of carnitine which aids fat utilization by muscles. Ensures adequate calcium absorption. Helps form collagen. Important for immune function.		Poor dietary intake of Lysine. High levels of Arginine. Connective tissue and bone disorders. High triglyceride levels. Viral infections (e.g. cold sores, shingles). Wrinkles. Decreased muscle mass. Cardiovascular disease - high serum triglycerides. Osteoporosis.	Lysine carnitine	Impaired Lysine metabolism. Vitamins B3 and B6 are required for metabolism of Lysine. Impaired metabolism of Lysine.	Vitamin C, Niacin, Vitamin B6, Iron, α-Ketoglutarate, Iron	Poultry, meats, fish, beans (esp. Soy), milk, cheese, egg, grains, cereals (esp. Oatmeal), gelatin, some vegetables (esp. White potato, green peas, asparagus, broccoli, corn, mushrooms and spinach), avocado, wheat germ,

Interpretation of Amino Acid Analysis

Amino Acid	Properties	Biosynthesis	Low	Treatment	High	Treatment	Food Sources
Methionine *essential sulphur amino acid*	Aids in increasing growth hormone production antioxidant and has detoxifying properties Assists the breakdown of fats Helps diminish muscle weakness Promotes the healthy metabolism of estrogen Reduces histamine levels in the body.	A precursor to the amino acids Cysteine and Taurine precursor to glutathione precursor to Creatine phosphate, an energy source for muscles	May cause adverse effects on sulphur metabolism Impaired phase II liver detoxification Methylation impairment Allergies Autism Brittle hair Cardiovascular disease Connective tissue and bone disorders Estrogen imbalances (low methylated estrogens); increased cancer risk Fatty liver Poor growth Muscle weakness Schizophrenia Undermethylation (Histapenia) Vascular dementia	Methionine Assess histamine levels Assess oxidative stress	excessive intake of Methionine-rich protein High Homocysteine levels Bone mineral loss Coronary artery disease Over methylation (Histadelia). Impaired phase II liver detoxification Folic acid deficiency (if 1-methylHistidine, 3-methylHistidine, cystathionine, Glycine, Histidine, Homocysteine, Methionine, sarcosine, or Serine are also elevated) Deficiency in cofactors required for Methionine to Cysteine and Taurine conversion (if Cysteine or Taurine are low).	Vitamin B6 α-Ketoglutarate Magnesium SAMe Me-Folate Assess histamine levels	Nuts, beef, lamb, cheese, turkey, pork, fish, shellfish, soy, egg, dairy, and beans, Cereals (e.g. Couscous, millet and oatmeal), Cottage cheese, grains

Amino Acid	Properties	Biosynthesis	Low	Treatment	High	Treatment	Food Sources
Ornithine	Key role in nitrogen metabolism. Involved in the release of growth hormones. Necessary for a healthy immune system.	Produced from Arginine in the urea cycle	Low Arginine levels. As a source of regulatory polyamines, a low level can affect cellular metabolism	Arginine	Adrenal fatigue. A block in the urea cycle (if elevated Glutamine or low glutamic acid). Vitamin B6 deficiency (if Alanine, alpha-aminoadipic acid, beta-Alanine, Aspartic acid, beta-aminoisobutyric acid, cystathione, Glycine, homocystine, Isoleucine, Leucine, Serine, Threonine, Tyrosine or Valine are also elevated). a possible metabolic block in urea cycle, causing excess ammonia burden. Confirm by checking for high Glutamine, low glutamic acid	Magnesium α-Ketoglutarate	

Interpretation of Amino Acid Analysis

Amino Acid	Properties	Biosynthesis	Low	Treatment	High	Treatment	Food Sources
Phenylalanine *essential amino acid*	Stimulates the secretion of gastrin	Precursor to Tyrosine precursor to dopamine, noradrenaline, adrenaline and thyroid hormones	Hyperinsulinemia (if Tyrosine is elevated) altered thyroid function and catecholamine deficits; depression, memory loss fatigue chronic stress autonomic dysfunction Arthritis Pain Poor memory Vitiligo Hyperinsulinemia (if Tyrosine is elevated)	Reduce lifestyle stressors Phenylalanine	Excessive protein intake iron, vitamin C, niacin - cofactors required for the conversion of Phenylalanine to Tyrosine phenylketonuria	Tyrosine (if indicated) Iron Vitamin C Niacin Low Phenylalanine diet	Soybeans, cheese, nuts, seeds, beef, lamb, chicken, pork, fish, egg, dairy, beans, and whole grains, Nuts & seeds Sweet potato Corn Green peas White potato Spinach Bananas
Phosphoethanolamine *Amino acid metabolite*	Precursor to synthesis of glycerophospholipid and the other a sphingomyelin used in cancer therapies				Zinc deficiency (if Phosphoserine is also elevated) Suspect parathyroid dysfunction (if Phosphoserine is also elevated) Methylation abnormality possible inhibition of choline and acetylcholine synthesis due to impaired Methionine metabolism involving methylation by S-adenosylmeth+ionine (SAM).	S-adenosyl-l-Methionine (SAMe) Vitamin Folate Betaine	

135

Alchemy of Amino Acids

Amino Acid	Properties	Biosynthesis	Low	Treatment	High	Treatment	Food Sources
Phosphoserine	Phospholipid and is a component of the cell membrane key role in cell signaling				Magnesium deficiency (if phosphoethanolamine is elevated relative to Serine) Suspect parathyroid dysfunction (if Phosphoserine is also elevated).	S-adenosyl-Methionine (SAMe) Vitamin Folate Betaine	
Proline *non-essential*	Collagen synthesis healthy immune system weak agonist of the Glycine receptor and of both NMDA and non-NMDA (AMPA/kainate) ionotropic Glutamate receptors. Used in brewing as an osmo-protectant	Synthesized from Glutamate Proline metabolized to AKG. Niacin (cofactor precursor) helps oxidize Proline to Glutamate.	Defective connective tissue synthesis Poor wound healing Wrinkles	α-Ketoglutarate	Connective tissue and bone disorders Poor wound healing Wrinkles Poor utilization of Proline A deficiency in the cofactors required for the conversion of Proline to Glutamate (e.g. niacin). May be genetic disorder associated with renal and CNS dysfunction	vitamin C to aid collagen synthesis Niacin Vitamin C	Asparagus, avocados, bamboo shoots, beans, brewer's yeast, broccoli rabe, brown rice bran, cabbage, caseinate, chives, dairy products, egg fish, lactalbumin, legumes, meat, nuts, seafood, seaweed, seeds, soy, spinach, watercress, whey, whole grains
Sarcosine (N-methylGlycine)	Intermediate of Glycine synthesis and degradation related compounds dimethylglycine (DMG) and trimethylglycine (TMG), is formed via the metabolism of nutrients such as choline and Methionine				Sarcosinemia can result from severe folate deficiency because of the folate requirement for the conversion of sarcosine to Glycine. Folic acid deficiency (if 1-methylHistidine, 3-methylHistidine, cystathionine, Glycine, Histidine, homocystine, Methionine, or Serine are also elevated) vitamin B2 deficiency	Vit B2 Folic acid	Egg yolks, turkey, ham, vegetables, legumes

Interpretation of Amino Acid Analysis

Amino Acid	Properties	Biosynthesis	Low	Treatment	High	Treatment	Food Sources
Serine *nonessential amino acid*	Needed for the proper metabolism of fats and fatty acids Contributes to a healthy immune system required for proper metabolism of Methionine	Produced endogenously from dietary Phosphoserine (magnesium dependent), Glycine and Threonine derived from glycolysis provided vitamin B6 and magnesium levels are adequate	Malabsorption Vitamin B6, folate and manganese deficiency (if Threonine is high) Disordered Methionine metabolism Deficits in acetylcholine metabolism elevated Homocysteine simultaneous high Threonine or Phosphoserine, then need for co-factors	Vitamin B6 Manganese Folic acid	Glucogenic compensation and catabolism (if Threonine is low) Vitamin B6 deficiency (if Alanine, alpha-aminoadipic acid, beta-Alanine, Aspartic acid, beta-aminoisobutyric acid, cystathione, Glycine, Homocysteine, Isoleucine, Leucine, Ornithine, Threonine, Tyrosine or Valine are also elevated) Folic acid deficiency (if 1-methylHistidine, 3-methylHistidine, cystathionine, Glycine, Histidine, Homocysteine, Methionine, sarcosine, or Serine are also elevated) Hyperinsulinemia (if Alanine or Glycine are also elevated). Glucogenic compensation and catabolism when accompanied by low Threonine, indicates glucogenic compensation and catabolism.	Threonine Vitamin B6 Folic acid	Dairy and meat, including certain cuts of pork, beef, elk, veal, bison, lamb, rabbit, deer, chicken, turkey, duck and goose, soy, peanuts

Amino Acid	Properties	Biosynthesis	Low	Treatment	High	Treatment	Food Sources
Taurine *semi-essential sulphur containing amino acid*	Stabilizes cell membranes in electrically active tissues, such as the brain and heart antioxidant and detoxifying properties production of bile. Females do not synthesize Taurine as easily as males.	Derived from Methionine and Cysteine	Oxidative stress Fat maldigestion High cholesterol Seizure disorders Cardiovascular disorders Arrhythmias Atherosclerosis Bile insufficiency Cardiovascular disease Chemical exposure and sensitivities Connective tissue and bone disorders Depression Fatigue High cholesterol Hypoglycemia Hypertension Macular degeneration Post viral or bacterial infections Xenobiotic exposure Seizure disorders Vegetarian diets. Vitamin B6 deficiency (if Taurine is low compared to cystine and/or Cysteine)	Taurine Cysteine Magnesium Vitamin B6	excessive inflammation Arrhythmias Cardiovascular disease Connective tissue and bone disorders. Fat maldigestion and fat soluble vitamin deficiency (if Taurine is elevated in the urinary sample only) Oxidative stress Impaired phase II liver detoxification Magnesium deficiency (if Taurine is elevated in the urinary sample only) Molybdenum deficiency Vitamin B6 deficiency, resulting in elevated beta-Alanine, which competes for Taurine renal conservation (if Leucine, isoleucine and Valine are also high) Wasting of Taurine (for urinary sample only).	Investigate causes for renal wasting (for high urinary Taurine) Vitamin E Vitamin C Beta-carotene CoQ10 Lipoate	Ice cream, cow's milk, shellfish, especially scallops, mussels, and clams. Dark meat of turkey and chicken, and turkey meat

Interpretation of Amino Acid Analysis

Amino Acid	Properties	Biosynthesis	Low	Treatment	High	Treatment	Food Sources
Threonine *essential amino acid*	Component of all connective tissue proteins (collagen, elastin, tooth enamel) Plays a key role in nitrogen metabolism Required in the formation of glycoproteins Necessary for a healthy immune system.	Precursor for Serine and Glycine metabolised to pyruvate and used as an energy source	Hypoglycemia particularly if Serine and Glycine are low Protein-deficient diet Malabsorption Manganese deficiency Rapid transit time. Decreased growth Decreased muscle mass	balanced or custom mixture of essential amino acids.	Excessive dietary intake Insufficient metabolism of Threonine Vitamin B6 deficiency (if Alanine, alpha-aminoadipic acid, beta-Alanine, Aspartic acid, beta-aminoisobutyric acid, cystathione, Glycine, homocystine, Isoleucine, Leucine, Ornithine, Serine, Tyrosine or Valine are also elevated)	Vitamin B6 Zinc.	Poultry, meats, fish, milk, beans (esp. Soy), cheese, egg, grains, nuts & seeds, cereals, gelatin, some vegetables (corn, green peas, white potato and spinach)
Tryptophan *essential amino acid*	Contributes to a healthy immune system Involved in growth hormone release	Precursor for serotonin, melatonin and niacin	Adrenal stress (if Arginine and Tyrosine are also low). Autism Depression Insomnia Mental health conditions Migraines Schizophrenia Sleep disorders.	Adrenal support phosphatidylserine magnesium vitamin C) 5-HTP	Inadequate metabolism of Tryptophan A deficiency in the cofactors required for the metabolism of Tryptophan (e.g. niacin, vitamin B6). possibly inadequate metabolism of Tryptophan	Niacin Vitamin B6	Meats, poultry, fish, beans (esp. Soy), milk, cheese, egg, grains, cereals, nuts & seeds, spirulina

Alchemy of Amino Acids

Amino Acid	Properties	Biosynthesis	Low	Treatment	High	Treatment	Food Sources
Tyrosine *nonessential amino acid*	Is iodinated to form the thyroid hormones. Aids in the production of melanin (the pigment responsible for hair and skin color). Supports the adrenal, thyroid, and pituitary glands.	Derived from Phenylalanine precursor in the synthesis of dopa, dopamine, norepinephrine and epinephrine (adrenaline)	Maldigestion Depression - Dopamine, noradrenaline and adrenaline imbalances Thyroid hormone imbalances Adrenal stress (if Arginine and Tryptophan are also low) A block in the conversion of Phenylalanine to Tyrosine Anxiety Behavioural and learning disorders Blood pressure disorders Inability to deal with stress Low sex drive Thyroid conditions.	Iron Tyrosine Vitamin C Niacin	inadequate utilization of Tyrosine. Attention deficit hyperactivity disorder (ADHD) Autism Blood pressure disorders Depression Schizophrenia Thyroid conditions. If Phenylalanine is normal or high (barring PKU), iron, vitamin C, and niacin supplementation might be indicated to help convert Phenylalanine to Tyrosine. Manganese deficiency (if Alanine, Isoleucine, Leucine or Valine are also elevated) Deficiencies in cofactors needed for Tyrosine metabolism (e.g. iron, vitamin B6, vitamin C).	Vitamin C Vitamin B6 Cu Iron	Poultry, meats, fish, beans (esp. Soy), cheese, egg, milk, grains, cereals (esp. Oatmeal and couscous), some vegetables (corn, white potato and spinach), nuts & seeds.

Interpretation of Amino Acid Analysis

Amino Acid	Properties	Biosynthesis	Low	Treatment	High	Treatment	Food Sources
Valine *essential amino acid*	Needed for muscle metabolism and tissue repair. Plays a key role in nitrogen metabolism		muscle loss. check for adequate HCl Maldigestion or leaky gut Bone and connective tissue disorders (if Isoleucine or Leucine are also low and hydroxyproline are elevated) Muscle atrophy. High alcohol intake Poor growth Catabolism of skeletal muscle	Digestive support (e.g. HCl, Digestive enzymes, L-Glutamine, Probiotics)	Excessive amino acid or Valine intake Vitamin B6 deficiency Manganese deficiency (if Alanine, alpha-aminoadipic acid, Isoleucine, Leucine, or Tyrosine are also elevated)	Vitamin B6 Check for insulin resistance.	Poultry, meats, fish, milk, cheese, egg, beans (esp. Soy), grains, nuts & seeds, cereals (esp. In millet, buckwheat groats, oatmeal), some vegetables (white potato, sweet potato, broccoli, corn, green peas, spinach and swiss chard), avocado, chocolate.

Urine amino acid laboratory result

Laboratory results may vary in appearance and style but will report the level of each amino acid. Creatinine is measured as a concentration reference point.

INTEGRATIVE MEDICINE

URINE, 24 HOUR	Result	Range	Units
Total Branched Chain AAs	311 *L	424 - 557	umol/L
GABA	<1.0	0.0 - 1.0	mmol/molCr
Hydroxylysine	2.2	2.0 - 5.0	umol/L
AMINO ACIDS, Urine.			
24hr Urine Volume	3250	693 - 3741	mL
Creatinine Concentration	1385.0	600.0 - 2000.0	mg/24hr
Specimen Validity			
24hr Urinary Ammonia	34200	11000 - 60000	umol/24h
Glutamine/Glutamate	0.3 *L	5.0 - 160.0	RATIO
Taurine, Urine	88.3 *H	16.0 - 80.0	mmol/molC
Threonine, Urine	<1.0 *L	7.0 - 29.0	mmol/molC
Valine, Urine	1.8 *L	3.0 - 13.0	mmol/molC
Cysteine, Urine	<1.0 *L	3.0 - 17.0	mmol/molC
Methionine, Urine	2.1	2.0 - 16.0	mmol/molC
Isoleucine, Urine	1.9	0.0 - 4.0	mmol/molCr
Leucine, Urine	<1.0 *L	2.0 - 11.0	mmol/molC
Phenylalanine, Urine	<1.0 *L	2.0 - 19.0	mmol/molC
Histidine, Urine	23.8 *L	26.0 - 153	mmol/molC
Tryptophane, Urine	<1.0	0.0 - 7.0	mmol/molCr
Arginine, Urine	<1.0	0.0 - 5.0	mmol/molCr
Lysine, Urine	10.1	7.0 - 58.0	mmol/molC
Aspartate, Urine	1.3 *L	2.0 - 7.0	mmol/molC
Hydroxyproline, Urine	<1.0	< 13.0	mmol/molCr
Serine, Urine	<1.0 *L	21.0 - 50.0	mmol/molC
Asparagine, Urine	<1.0	0.0 - 23.0	mmol/molCr
Glutamate, Urine	10.6	0.0 - 12.0	mmol/molCr
Glutamine, Urine	2.9 *L	20.0 - 76.0	mmol/molC
Proline, Urine	<1.00	0.00 - 9.00	mmol/molCr
Glycine, Urine	41.0 *L	43.0 - 173	mmol/molC
Alanine, Urine	10.2 *L	16.0 - 68.0	mmol/molC
Tyrosine, Urine	<1.0 *L	2.0 - 23.0	mmol/molC
Citrulline, Urine	<1.00	< 4.00	mmol/molCr
Ornithine, Urine	<1.0	< 5.0	mmol/molCr
1 Methyl Histidine, Urine	334 *H	< 40.0	mmol/molCr
3 Methyl Histidine, Urine	23.2	18.0 - 47.0	mmol/molC

(*) Result outside normal reference range   (H) Result is above upper limit of reference rang   (L) Result is below lower limit of reference range

Receiving the results of an amino acid analysis can be so exciting as it reveals imbalances in many organ systems.

1. Key features in interpreting amino acid results
2. Identify urine concentration and clearance through the assessment of creatinine and ammonia. **Creatinine** is a waste product excreted in the urine that comes from normal wear and tear of muscles. Creatinine values are a result of production driven by muscle mass and elimination driven by filtration in the kidneys.
3. Identifying **patterns of imbalance**. Groups of amino acids play a role in specific organ functions. For example, examine the levels of Methionine, Tryptophan, Tyrosine, Phenylalanine, Glycine and GABA for neurotransmitter production.
4. Crosscheck the patterns of amino acid imbalance with the chart the end of this chapter. This will reveal organ systems that may need attention and treatment.
5. Examine and identify imbalances of each individual amino acid, what is meant to have higher or a lower level, how does this imbalance affect the physiology, what are the corrective measures, and where is it found in the diet.

Once identified, formulate a custom compounded amino acid blend personalized for the individual based on your finding. Refer to custom compounding of amino acids. You may wish to consult with a compounding pharmacist for further guidance.

Please view interpretation of amino acids in **Alchemy of Amino Acids Masterclass**.

Let's have a peak the interpretation of some results.

Case 1

Adult male with hypertension and tachycardia.

Diet mainly vegetarian.

Results:

HIGH	LOW	
	▲	**Isoleucine**
	▲	**Leucine**
	▲	**Taurine**
▲		**Methionine**

Low Taurine level with high normal Methionine indicates a problem with the pathway from Homocysteine to Taurine.

Support low Taurine with addition of co-factor, Vit B6 and Taurine. If Taurine remains low, consider a genetic impairment thus requiring sustained Taurine supplementation.

Low Leucine and Isoleucine is indicative of poor BCAA levels, poor muscle tone. Supplement with BCAA with Taurine and Vit B6.

Check methylation SAMe pathway for MTR, MTRR and AHCY mutations and support pathways with methylation co-factors.

Case 2

Adult male with depression, occasional recreational drug user.

HIGH	LOW	
	▲	**Histamine**
▲		**Phenylalanine**
▲		**Tyrosine**

Elevated Tyrosine level may be associated with bronchospasm and impaired PO2. Support conversion of Tyrosine to Adrenaline, the chief bronchodilator typically used in anaphylaxis with Vitamin C and Copper, cofactors of dopamine carboxylation.

Copper and Vit C supplementation may reduce bronchospasm. Supplement with Histadine, Copper and Vit B6 to support dopamine decarboxylase, the conversion from Dopamine to catecholamines.

Case 3

Schizophrenia patient with anxiety and sleep disorders.

HIGH	LOW	
	▲	**Lysine**
	▲	**Valine**
	▲	**Leucine**
	▲	**Isoleucine**
	▲	**Glycine**
	▲	**Serine**

Low Lysine and low BCAA's is associated with anxiety. Elevated levels of fatty acid organic acid metabolites are indicative of carnitine deficiency, a shuttle for fatty acid transport into mitochondria for energy production.

Low Glycine and Serine are associated with poor sleep onset and maintenance of sleep.

Consider carnitine supplementation to help metabolic demand for energy production from fatty acid oxidation. Supplement with Lysine, Glycine, Serine and free-form amino acids (base formula).

Case 4

Anxiety and sleep disorder

HIGH	LOW	
	▲	**Lysine (VERY LOW)**
	▲	**Phenylalanine**

Lysine deficiency is a possible moderator of Serotonin hypersensitivity and associated with anxiety, sleep disturbances and IBS.

Supplement with Lysine, Phenylalanine and Tyrosine for management of anxiety.

Add Glycine and Theanine to support GABA production and anxiety management.

Case 5

Anxiety, insomnia, panic, disturbed sleep maintenance in a young male.

HIGH	LOW	
	▲	**GABA**
	▲	**Glutamine**
	▲	**Ornithine**
	▲	**Serine**
	▲	**Glycine**

Sleep architecture has been shown to improve with supplementation of Ornithine, Glycine and Serine. For anxiety, supplement with Theanine, GABA and Glycine.

Case 6

Young male with behavioral problems and addiction to marijuana.

HIGH	LOW	
▲		**Histamine**
▲		**Asparagine**
▲		**Glutamine**

All three amino acids are high which reflects possible defect in SN-1 and SN-2 transporter systems.

Supplement with Methionine, Tyrosine and GABA. Give Magnesium and B-group vitamins as essential co-factors for amino acid transamination.

Case 7

Elderly man with major cognitive failure, poor memory, loss of focus and walk is shuffled.

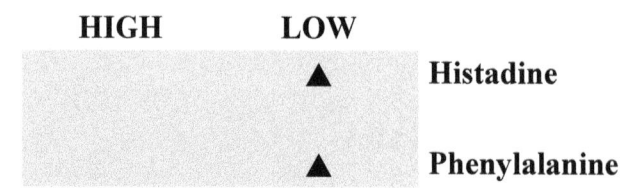

HIGH	LOW	
	▲	**Histadine**
	▲	**Phenylalanine**

Supplement with 5-HTP

Stimulation of Histadine conversion to Histamine leads to depleted total body Histadine. Low Histadine levels affects the brain and immune system leading to metabolic stress due to histamine insufficiency. Check Iron studies as low hematocrit and low hemoglobin could further deplete Histamine.

Case 8

Adult female with adrenal fatigue and diagnosis of chronic fatigue syndrome.

HIGH	LOW	
▲		**Arginine**
▲		**Ornithine**

High Arginine would potentially block the urea cycle especially if urea is low and Glutamine, Citrulline, or Ornithine is also elevated. Consider a carefully controlled low protein diet to regulate ammonemia.

Supplement with co-factor Manganese if Arginine is elevated in comparison to Ornithine, Magnesium and Alpha-keto-glutarate.

Elevations in Ornithine is associated with adrenal fatigue representing a potential block in the urea cycle particularly if Glutamine is elevated or Glutamic Acid is depleted.

Case 9
Anxiety, allergies, fatigue

HIGH	LOW	
▲		Histamine
▲		GABA
▲		Aspartic
▲		Glutamine
▲		Ornithine
	▲	Citrulline

Elevations in Ornithine exhibits manifestations of Ornithine trans carbamylase (OCT) deficiency. Glutamine and Aspartic Acid are extremely elevated indicating general metabolic acidosis with nitrogen transport impairment.

Many other amino acids are in their high normal and moderately elevated ranges. The passage of Histamine, Glutamine and Aspartic Acid into the urine keep their blood levels within normal limits.

Ornithine is a primary urea cycle intermediate which indicates a metabolic backup due to lack of urea cycle activity.

Stimulate metabolism with exercise, low protein diet high complex carbohydrate diet, and co-factors, namely Magnesium, alpha-ketoglutarate, zinc and B-group vitamins.

Case 10

Recurrent UTI, interstitial cystitis followed by immune dysregulation. Respiratory infection, body aches.

HIGH	LOW	
	▲	**Glutamic acid**
	▲	**Glutamine**

Low Glutamate is associated with metabolic fragility because of difficulty in responding to systemic pH and ammonia.

Bladder infections and general body pain tends to be worse in the morning, a time when systemic pH is under stress from stimulation of cortisol release and ammonia formation.

Low Glutamine may be associated with renal acidosis due to increased renal glutaminase activity and increased ammonia excretion, a form of negative nitrogen balance.

If ammonia toxicity is confirmed, use a low protein, high complex carbohydrate diet with supplementation of Vit B6, α-ketoglutarate branch chain amino acids.

Correlation between organ system imbalance with amino acid patterns

Suspect a health condition if you see high's or low's of certain amino acids.

Gastro-intestinal	
Leaky gut if:	Elevated Anserine, Carnosine & low (or low normal) essential AAs (dietary peptides)
	Low Leucine, Isoleucine, Valine
	Rule out pancreatic dysfunction, zinc deficiency
Fat maldigestion if:	Low or elevated (urine only) Taurine or Glycine (needed for bile salt production)
	Rule out deficiency of fat-soluble nutrients
Intestinal malabsorption if:	Low Threonine and other essential AA's

GIT & Detox	
Intestinal dysbiosis if:	Elevated gamma-aminobutyric acid, alpha-aminoadipic acid, beta-Alanine, ethanolamine or ammonia (may be produced by intestinal bacteria or yeast)
Impaired ammonia detoxication if:	Elevated Glutamine with elevated Arginine or Citrulline or Ornithine and low urea (impaired urea cycle)
	Elevated ammonia with high urea suggests protein overload
	Elevated ammonia with high ammonia concentration and normal urea suggests decayed specimen
	Alpha ketoglutarate (1.5 to 3g/day)

Detoxification	
Impaired hepatic detoxication if:	Elevated or low Methionine, Cysteine, cystathionine, Taurine (suggestive of impaired phase 2 methylation, sulfation) Elevated beta Alanine (may lead to Taurine deficiency) Low Glycine, Glutamine, Aspartic acid (utilized in Phase 2 detoxication) Supplement with amino acids, vitamin B6, B12, folic acid or betaine as needed
Cardiovascular	
Increased susceptibility to occlusive arterial disease if:	Elevated Homocysteine Low cystathionine low Methionine, Cysteine or Taurine Supplement with magnesium, vitamin B6, B12, folic acid, Serine, or betaine as needed (to facilitate Methionine metabolism)
Musculoskeletal	
Increased risk of collagen or inflammation:	Elevated Homocysteine with low cystathionine Homocysteine interferes with crosslinking of collagen Elevated or low cyst(e)ine, Taurine Low Methionine, Lysine, Low Leucine, Isoleucine, Valine Elevated Hydroxyproline and Proline, 3-methylHistidine (suggestive of tissue catabolism) Elevated Anserine, carnosine (suggestive of poor tissue regeneration) Supplement with magnesium, vitamin B6, B12, folic acid, betaine as needed. Ensure adequate zinc

Interpretation of Amino Acid Analysis

Neurological

Neurological / behavioral problems if:	Elevated or low Tryptophan, Taurine, Phenylalanine, Tyrosine (NT precursors) Elevated (or normal) Homocysteine, with elevated or low Methionine & low cystathionine (suggestive of low SAME), low Taurine, low B6 Supplement with vitamin B6 and B12 Ensure adequacy of zinc, riboflavin, magnesium (all needed for B6 activation)

Endocrine

Adrenal insufficiency if:	Low Alanine (increased conversion of Alanine to pyruvate) Elevated Ornithine (weakness of Ornithine transaminase)
Adrenal hyperactivity if:	Elevated Alanine (increased conversion from pyruvate) Low Arginine, Tryptophan, Tyrosine (upregulation of arginase)
Hyperinsulinemia if:	Low Phenylalanine (upregulated conversion to Tyrosine) Elevated Serine, Alanine, Glycine (gluconeogenic amino acids)
Suspect parathyroid dysfunction if:	Elevated Phosphoserine with elevated phosphoethanolamine Assess cortisol and DHEA levels
Oxidative Stress	Significantly elevated cystine, compared to Cysteine (urine only) (cystine is the oxidized form of Cysteine) Low cyst(e)ine (plasma or urine) (Cysteine necessary for glutathione production) Low or elevated (urine only) Taurine (Taurine scavenges hypochlorite ions) Antioxidant support as needed Rule out magnesium deficiency

Nutrient Adequacy	
Suspect increased need for magnesium if:	Elevated ethanolamine, compared with phosphoethanolamine (conversion dependent upon Mg) Elevated Phosphoserine, compared with Serine (conversion dependent upon Mg) Low or elevated (urine only) Taurine (low Taurine causes body to waste Mg) Elevated Citrulline or Aspartic acid (conversions dependent upon Mg)

Treatment - Balancing Amino Acid levels

The joy of compounding nutrients personalized for an individual can be so rewarding as you can triturate doses, quality and potency of raw materials without any added adulterants such as colors, drying agents, flavors, preservatives, and stabilizing agents. Often, chronic complex inflammatory patients require a tailored amino acid therapy as they may be unable to tolerate the additives found in their medication.

The therapeutic benefit of taking a tailored amino acid blend can be experienced within hours of taking a dose. Amino acids are fundamental to life so they will reflect as optimization of physiological processes within the body.

Some might experience symptom relief right away, whereas others might not experience any change symptomatically for some time. Remember that amino acids are working intracellularly so the benefits might be experienced either immediately or over time.

Compounding an amino acid blend without any adulterants has limitations on stability and shelf life in accordance with compounding laws or pharmacy practice. It is for this reason, that amino acids are compounded individually for a patient based on the analysis at the time of dispensing only.

Take note of the characteristics of each amino acid during compounding. Some amino acids or granular or in a powder form, others are rather smelly, particularly the sulphur -containing amino acids, whereas, some may be hygroscopic or water loving which may render the entire blend unusable.

Amino acids work collaboratively with cofactors such as minerals and vitamins to support synthesis, metabolism and absorption. It is advisable to dispense a complex magnesium supplement with B-group vitamins with amino acids separately.

They may however, be taken in one collective dose together. Amino acids are best taken with water or juice before meals. If the powder compound is not palatable, you wish to add a natural flavoring agent. The powder compound can also be encapsulated by a compounding pharmacist for ease of dispensing and compliance.

Based on amino acid analysis and the clinical picture, certain amino acid derivatives or active ingredients may be added to the amino acid blend.

For example, AAKG, Arginine alpha ketoglutarate may be added to improve energy, endurance and enhance recovery as it regulates amino acid synthesis, energy production and the formation of free radicals.

The Amino Acids Analysis report details levels of amino acids based upon measured levels in blood plasma or urine. Supplement with amino acids that are in the low range at a triturated quantity depending on degree of depletion.

These levels are calculated based upon the measured level versus the reference range, the individual's age and sex, and a human needs tabulation derived from the National Research Council's table of amino acids requirements.

A custom-tailored amino acid supplement can be prescribed by your health practitioner and compounded by a compounding pharmacist or trained health care practitioner.

Custom compounded amino acids are formulated, compounded and dispensed in a homogenous powder to be taken orally with water or juice.

Take amino acids ideally a half hour before food with water or juice. If the formula does not dissolve easily, you may wish to dissolve the dose in a small amount of warm water then add the appropriate amount of water or juice.

Nutrient Co-factors

Because various vitamins and minerals are needed as cofactors in amino acid metabolism, abnormal patterns in blood or urine can provide telltale signs of functional deficiency of these nutrients.

Protein ingestion requires adequate levels of hydrochloric acid to initiate protein denaturation and stimulate pancreatic and biliary flow.

It is essential to optimize digestion either with amylase, lipase and protease supplementation. Manage hypochlorrhydria before considering amino acid therapy.

Abnormally low or high amino acid levels can be caused by dietary deficiencies of protein and micronutrients. Variations in metabolic demands by hormones or toxic factors could also increase the loss.

Amino acids that are subject to transamination can point to pyridoxal phosphate (vitamin B6) dysfunction. These include alpha-aminoadipic acid, Alanine, Aspartic acid, Tyrosine, Leucine, Isoleucine, and Valine.

Magnesium serves as an enzyme activator in a number of reactions, and certain elevations and deficits in amino acids can suggest a deficiency. The nutritional cofactors involved in amino acid metabolism include thiamine, riboflavin, niacin, B12 and folate, zinc, and manganese.

Vitamin B6 is the most important vitamin for amino acid transamination.

Cofactor need with Amino Acid imbalances

Supplement with Nutrients	Amino Acid Imbalances
Magnesium	Elevated ethanolamine, compared with phosphoethanolamine (conversion dependent upon Mg)
	Elevated Phosphoserine, compared with Serine (conversion dependent upon Mg)
	Low or elevated (urine only) Taurine (low Taurine causes body to waste Mg)
	Elevated Citrulline or Aspartic acid (conversions dependent upon Mg)
Iron	Elevated Phenylalanine (unless elevated Tyrosine, Tryptophan) - conversion dependent upon Fe
	Low Histidine (iron absorption dependent on HCl)
Manganese	Elevated Arginine, compared with Ornithine
	Elevated Alanine, alpha-aminoadipic acid, Tyrosine, Leucine, Isoleucine, or Valine (all are dependent upon alpha-ketoglutarate which depends upon isocitrate dehydrogenase, a Mn-dependent enzyme)
	Low Histidine (hypochlorhydria from deficient Histamine, may lead to Mn malabsorption)
	Low Threonine (suggests general malabsorption)

Zinc	Elevated Anserine, Carnosine (peptidases require zinc)
	Elevated phosphoethanolamine with elevated Phosphoserine
	Elevated Leucine, Isoleucine and Valine (Branched-chain amino acid peptidases require zinc)
Molybdenum	Elevated Taurine (with normal beta-Alanine)
	Elevated cyst(e)ine (with normal Lysine and Ornithine)
Vitamin B6	Elevated Cystathionine, Homocystine, Serine, Tyrosine, alpha-aminoadipic acid, beta-Alanine, Alanine, Threonine, Ornithine, Glycine, Aspartic acid, beta-aminoisobutyric acid, Leucine, Isoleucine, Valine
	Low Cysteine (compared with cystathionine) or low Taurine

Amino Acid Therapy

Information about individual amino acids may shed light to clinical responses to therapy. Patients who cannot sustain normal levels of amino acids in a fasting plasma may be candidates for individualized amino acid therapy.

Each amino acid has its own property, structure, function, synthesis, therapeutic use, dosage, and contra-indication.

Biochemical individuality demands selective use of amino acid supplements for each patient.

Ensuring a balanced and optimal intake nutrient co-factors and amino acids becomes critical for prevention as well as treatment of many chronic illnesses.

Amino acids are best absorbed if they are taken in L-isomer forms or in tri-peptides. In the case of Methionine and Phenylalanine, the DL form may be beneficial for its individual therapeutic need.

BCAA's are essential amino acids as they constitute about 35% of muscle tissue and need to be supplemented as they cannot be produced or synthesized by the body.

Large containers of protein powders are really popular in the exercise and sport industry. Most these agents contain BCAA's which are aimed specifically to:

- Increase muscle growth
- Increase stamina & endurance
- Increase fat burn
- Improve recovery & performance

Amino acids may be formulated with high levels of complex carbohydrates ideally for debilitated, malnourished or palliative care patients to provide sufficient nutrients in the healing and nourishing process.

Amino acid custom compound blends, specially compounded, are a blend of specific amino acids only based on lab results.

Amino Acids Vs Protein Powder

What's the difference between a custom compounded amino acid and commercially available protein powders for sport nutrition?

Huge tubs of protein powders have become a substantial and lucrative industry for the sports, weight loss and palliative industry.

Most sport protein formulae contain a blend of BCAA's – Leucine, Isoleucine, and Valine blended together with enhanced or activated amino acids such as AAKG, (Arginine alpha ketoglutarate), or Creatine to name a few, key players in amino acid metabolism.

Commercial amino acid formulae may contain vitamins, minerals, bulking agents, flavours, and colors to improve palatability and compliance.

Amino acid concentrations may vary based on:
- Source e.g. pea protein or whey protein
- Source variability – protein from the same plant animal source, climate, location, agricultural processes, location, transit time
- Isomer configuration extraction methods

Protein powders made from milk-derived whey and casein, egg white or soy protein are sources of quality protein that contain all the essential amino acids.

L-Glutamate (more commonly known as "MSG") is produced by bacterial fermentation. Creatine monohydrate supplements are manufactured outside the body from sarcosine and cyanamide (do not confuse with cyanide). They are generally combined in a reactor with other catalyst compounds.

Commercially available protein powders are usually vary in potency. The exact composition of amino acids in a specific source may vary depending on the location or breed of the source.

Protein composition derived from a whey source in a cow in New Zealand may differ from that of Europe even if the extraction methods are standardized.

Custom tailored amino acids are pure amino acids - no additives. – without any adulterants. It is recommended that supplementation of a good B complex with your amino-acid complex is optimal for its effectiveness.

Where do amino acids for supplementation come from?

Amino acids are derived from direct chemical synthesis, fermentation, and bio-conversion using enzymes chosen by manufacturers based on their specific technology, costs of raw material, market prices, market sizes, cost variances between processes, and environmental impacts.

Chemical synthesis or chemical extraction is the most common and cost-effective amino production process. The starting material for this process may be derived from animal by products high in keratin.

Keratin is a fibrous protein extremely high in amino acid concentrations. The highest amounts of keratin is primarily found in the hair, stratum corneum (outermost layer of skin), horns, nails, claws and hooves of mammals.

Fermentation uses enzymes combined with vegetables such as corn or sugarcane to extract the amino acids. The corn/sugar cane is broken down into glucose which then ferments with various enzymes.

The fermented result goes through a cellular separation process, crystallization process, and crystal separation process before being dried, weighed, and packaged. The varying steps to this process and utilization of inconsistent plant bases creates variances from batch to batch.

Corn offers a higher quality and more cost-effective alternative – fermented vegan BCAAs. These are usually manufactured in Japan or Korea and are derived mainly from corn and other grains.

Fermented vegan BCAAs, or any fermented amino acids, for that matter, tend to taste much better and may have a slight sour taste.

Another source of amino acids is low-allergenic organic brown rice protein concentrate, extracted by natural enzymes at low temperature from the wholegrain, including the bran, germ and endosperm. This unique process produces a smooth texture that mixes easily

Organic whole grain brown rice protein (98%), organic whole grain rice milk powder, enzymes, vegetable gum (xanthan gum), sweetener (steviol glycosides, thaumatin), flavor (vanilla and caramel).

Amino Acid concentrations in Different types of Protein sources

Treatment – Balancing Amino Acid levels

The composition of amino acids may vary based on primary sources. A glutamate toxic patient would be best to choose an amino acid supplement from a pea source based on composition of amino acids in each source.

Amino Acid	Whey Isolate	Pea Protein	Soy Isolate	Brown Rice Protein
Alanine	4.8%	4.2%	4.3%	5.6%
Arginine	1.8	8.7	7.5	8.3
Aspartate (Aspartic acid)	10.2	11.5	11.8	8.8
Cysteine	2.1	16.1	1.2	2.4
Glutamate (glutamic acid)	19.5	3.1	18.9	18.5
Glycine	1.4	4.2	4.2	4.3
Histidine	1.3	2.1	2.6	2.4
Isoleucine *	5.6	4.8	4.8	4.0
Leucine *	10.3	8.3	8.2	8.5
Lysine *	9.7	7.3	6.3	2.8
Methionine *	1.7	1.0	1.2	2.8
Phenylalanine*	2.6	5.3	5.2	5.4
Proline	5.7	4.5	5.0	4.8
Serine	4.9	5.1	5.2	5.1
Threonine *	7.9	4.0	3.7	3.7
Tryptophan *	1.9	1.0	1.3	1.3
Tyrosine	2.7	3.8	3.7	5.4
Valine *	5.9	5.0	4.9	5.9

- Amino acids marked * are regarded as being essential dietary requirements, i.e. they cannot be manufactured by the body, and therefore must be consumed on a regular basis. All the other amino acids are classed as non-essential, as the body is able to synthesize them from various substrates.
- The total BCAA content of these four protein sources are 21.8%, 18.1%, 17.9% and 18.4% respectively.

- Figures are listed as a percentage of total amino acid content for each product.
- Figures are derived from product information provided by product suppliers.
- Each manufacturer provides protein powders with differing total concentrations of amino acids per 100g of powder. With rice protein for example, this may be as low as 626g/kg, whereas for pea protein isolates, the amino acid content may vary from 69 – 84%, depending on the product.

Compounding Amino Acids

Features of amino acids may vary based on density, solubility, coarseness and taste. The density of amino acids vary in that a scoop of one amino acid may weigh 3g whereas another may weigh 2g.

Features of Amino acids

A well-known property possessed by amino acids is their ability to combine with acids and with bases. However, some amino acids have hygroscopic characteristics in that they absorb water rendering the entire complex oxidized and damaged. Choline and Cysteine are examples of hygroscopic amino acids.

The density of each amino acid varies. Ensure that you follow the compounding guidelines to ensure that you supply the correct dose and blend consistently.

Weight is based on a level metric teaspoon rounded to nearest 0.5g.

Tasting are described on a consensus basis, away from food. This guide is an approximation only as materials can vary between batches according to milling and manufacture method as well as conditions such as humidity.

Tips for Best results

Most amino acids are thought to be absorbed best when taken on an empty stomach between meals and in divided doses.

However, there are always exceptions to the rule and there may also be several co factors that are required for the uptake of amino acids which will be listed.

- Most amino acids will be well tolerated by the general population. Some individuals however, can experience stomach upsets and nausea which dictates that these amino acids may be taken with meals, although this is said to reduce absorption and uptake in cells due to the competitiveness of other amino acids.
- Store in a cool, dry area away from light
- Some health practitioners may dose with a single amino acid for a specific condition. It is advisable to dose for a limited time
- A custom compounded amino acid blend may be taken for as long the body needs it. Dose 3 to 5 g twice a day for 3 months, then reassess with an amino acid analysis to establish the need for ongoing treatment, dose adjustment or cessation
- Amino acids are usually compounded for chronic and complex conditions

General information on free form

L, DL, Acetyl form - amino acid bioavailability

Unlike protein meals or protein powders, Crystalline, or free form amino acids, are absorbed into the bloodstream and available to tissues within 20 minutes of ingestion, requiring no digestive processes for absorption.

- Amino acids compete for uptake into the body. They are most efficacious when taken under the tongue on an empty stomach where they are then absorbed directly into the bloodstream. Alternatively, using a pure carbohydrate in the form of fruit or juice to help wash them down is also effective, particularly when wanting to transport a free form amino acid into the brain.

- All protein foods are made up of amino acids, so if a free form amino acid needs to be taken with food because of nausea concerns, and/or for convenience, chose a carbohydrate food or liquid. Otherwise, allow at least 20 mins before a meal or ingesting another amino acid
- Only the Acetyl form of amino acid passively travels to the brain through the blood brain barrier (BBB) unaided; the free form amino acids need to be actively carried through and competition to the brain from other amino acids is fierce. The amino acids Tryptophan, Tyrosine, Phenylalanine and Inositol are very competitive with each other.
- Research suggests amino acids are more receptive to muscle tissue post exercise when nutrient uptake is enhanced by increased blood flow

L Arginine HCL:

Tips for GH production

L-Arginine, or l-Arginine hydrochloride, taken on an empty stomach, will cause a significant release of growth hormone in many people.

L-Arginine is most effective as a growth hormone releaser for people between the ages of about 25 to 45.

It is necessary, however, to use a very large dose of Arginine: 10 to 30 g, depending upon many factors such as one's age and body weight.

Treatment – Balancing Amino Acid levels

Amino Acid	Weight	Solubility	Textures	Texture	Taste
L-Arginine	3000	*	VF	fine salt	bitter
Acetyl L-Carnitine	2000	**	VF	fine salt	sour
L-Carnitine	2500	***	VF	Salt	lemon
L-Choline	3000	***s	VF	fine salt	tangy
L-Citrulline	2000	*	VF	corn flour	sour
N-Acetyl L-Cysteine	3500	**	VF	Crystalline	sour/sulphur
N-Acetyl D-Glucosamine	1500	***		icing sugar	sweet
Gamma Amino Butyric Acid	3000	***	VF	fine salt	neutral
L-Glucosamine	3000	***		Corn flour	sweet
L-Glutamine	2500	*	VF	flour	earthy
Glycine	3500	***	VF	sugar	extra sweet
Inositol	3000	***	VF	icing sugar	sweet
L-Lysine	3000	**	VF	granular	neutral
L-Methionine	2000	*	VF	fine grains	bitter/sulphur
L-Ornithine	2500	***	VF	corn flour	neutral
L-Phenylalanine	2500	*	VF	flour	bitter
L-Proline	2000	*	VF	icing sugar	sweet
Taurine	3000	**s	VF	crystalline	bitter
L-Theanine	2000	***	VF	icing sugar	neutral
L-Threonine	2500	**	VF	corn flour	neutral
L-Tryptophan	1000	*	VF	corn flour	bitter
L-Tyrosine	2000	*	VF	corn flour	neutral

Solubility Guide: *Low **Med ***High | VF: Vegan Friendly | S: ≤ 1% silica

Tips for effectiveness

Arginine levels can best be maintained by not taking it continuously. A schedule of something like four weeks of continuous use followed by a two-week break generally works best.

When carbohydrates are present in large amounts, particularly when combined with high temperatures (like post workout), it can be rendered nutritionally unavailable to the body, so take well away from carbohydrate-based meals.

Acetyl L Carnitine

Best time of day to take Acetyl L- Carnitine:

Best taken in the morning before breakfast. Add Alpha Lipoic acid for heart health.

L Carnitine bi tartrate

Tips for Absorption

Absorption is the key for maximum effects in fat loss. Insulin is the most effective agent at helping more L-carnitine get inside muscle cells. So, by combining L-carnitine with an insulin elevating supplement or meal, you can ensure maximum carnitine retention in muscle cells.

Best time of day to take L-Carnitine

It all depends on your primary goal. If your main concern is fat loss, then it's best to take carnitine with your largest meals of the day. If your primary goal is muscle growth, performance, or recovery, then you're best to take carnitine before and after your workouts with some insulin-spiking carbs

An effective dosage of L-carnitine tartrate is 1,000 to 2,000 millig daily, usually split up into two serving

L Choline bi tartrate

Tips for Fat Loss

For fat loss, take pre or post exercise on an empty stomach.

Choline works by lipolysis, so best taken during the day.

Tips for Brain Function

Choline bitartrate is difficult to convert to Acetyl Choline in the brain, but some people have found success using choline bitartrate to promote lucid dreaming and enhance REM sleep. Even using choline for this purpose, it is better to take during the day as Choline at night is known to keep some people awake.

L Citrulline Malate

Tips for stacking with Arginine

Citrulline Malate may be taken to increase the effectiveness of Arginine supplementation as Citrulline bypasses the processes that convert Arginine to NO within the liver.

Consider taking Citrulline Malate and Arginine 20 mins apart for optimum plasma levels of Arginine. Doses over 5g of Citrulline Malate may cause stomach upsets.

N-Acetyl Cysteine

Special tips

Regular supplementation with NAC will increase the urinary excretion of copper. If using NAC for an extended period of time, it's probably wise to add both copper (2 mg a day) and zinc (30 mg a day) to your treatment regimen.

If you use NAC for more than a month, add a mixed amino acid complex to your treatment regimen to ensure that you are getting adequate, balanced amounts of all the Amino acids.

Tips for absorption of NAC

NAC is most effective when taken on an empty stomach, with a small amount of vitamin C powder mixed in.

If you've added a mixed amino acid complex to your NAC regimen, be sure to take it on an empty stomach as well, but at a different time of day than you take the NAC.

As the Acetyl portion of the amino acid is quite irritating to the teeth, taking it through a straw is advised, and it also makes it more palatable

Special caution

Evidence indicates that in some healthy individuals, high doses of NAC (3,000 mg a day) can act as a pro-oxidant rather than an antioxidant, actually lowering levels of glutathione rather than increasing them.

For this reason, otherwise healthy individuals may want to avoid taking high doses of NAC until more information is available.

N Acetyl D Glucosamine HCL

May be taken together with Threonine, Glutamine and Glycine for gut repair, celiac treatment and/or ulcerative colitis. Is heat stable.

Glucosamine HCL

Absorption

83% HCL VS 63% Sulphate, HCL is the original form of glucosamine. May be taken with or without food, but high doses are not to be taken (anything over 1500mg) by diabetics. May be taken with food.

L Glutamine

Tips for absorption for stomach ailments

Take it three times a day in divided doses on an empty stomach as it is sensitive to stomach acids

The best times to take it are in the morning, after a workout and before going to bed. Taking Glutamine when you wake up is ideal because your muscles have gone all night without nutrition.

Tips for absorption for sports performance

Taking it after a workout helps the muscles recover.

Taking it before bed helps increase growth hormone in your body.

Glycine

Best time to take Glycine

Though Glycine can be absorbed from food, it would be difficult on an ordinary diet to absorb enough to saturate the blood. At saturation levels, Glycine readily crosses the blood brain barrier via passive diffusion.

A supplemental dose of 3 g before bed readily accomplishes this.

For Creatine conversion

Glycine is best taken away from meals or pre-workout particularly if you would like to encourage conversion to Creatine.

Inositol

Tips for Anxiety/OCD treatment

If you take Inositol for anxiety/OCD, medical professionals advise starting with 2g twice a day. After one week, this can be increased to three times per day.

During the third week, you can slowly begin to increase the Inositol by small amounts to 3g three times daily; the fourth week, to 4,000 mg three times per day; and the fifth week, 5g three times each day. In the sixth week, you will reach a suggested maximum dosage of 6g three times a day.

You may find that using Inositol on its own may not be enough to treat anxiety. Many take it in conjunction with Omega-3 supplement, valerian root, and passionflower to enhance the effects.

There are a few side effects to watch out for when taking this supplement, although stomach upsets may occur, but studies have shown this to be a relatively normal side effect.

Some users report that their appetites greatly increased after starting an Inositol regime

There is some evidence to show that caffeine interferes with Inositol uptake.

Best time to take Inositol

There is conflicting evidence whether this amino acid can be taken all at once, in divided doses, with or without food, but it seems best absorbed in the morning before breakfast.

Inositol does not dissolve very well, so it needs to be stirred, and drunk while the water is still in motion.

L Lysine

L Lysine has no known toxicity. A few cases of abdominal cramps and diarrhea have been reported with very high doses (more than 10 g a day).

Best way to take Lysine

If you feel a virus coming on, take 1 Lysine every hour for 8 hours or until symptoms desist. Lysine is best taken on an empty stomach - but if you have forgotten a serving, you may take it with food.

Postmenopausal women can take Lysine with meals to encourage absorption of calcium by the body.

For cold sores: Take 1g L-Lysine three times a day with meals for flare-ups. If you are subject to recurrent outbreaks of cold sores, continue on a maintenance dosage of 1g per day.

L Methionine

Tips for absorption

During Methionine supplementation, intake of Taurine, Cysteine, and other sulphur containing amino acids, as well as B6 and folic acid should also be included. Taking it with a tablet for liver support would be ideal.

Recommended dosage of L-Methionine

Dosage ranges from 500 mg to 4g in divided dosages throughout the day, away from meals

Remember that those with high Homocysteine should only take 2 g a day

L Ornithine

Best time to take for performance

Studies show Ornithine reduces ammonia concentrations in the blood and thus enhances performance of prolonged exercise (45 minutes or more) which is in part due to Ornithine remaining elevated in the blood for a few hours after ingestion. On this basis, it is suggested pre-workout or between meals for reducing excess ammonia.

Best time to take when on a parasite treatment program

For parasites or in combination with Arginine (2 Arginine: 1 Ornithine ratio) for GH production, take before bed on an empty stomach.

L Phenylalanine

Special tips

With high blood pressure, start with very low amounts, such as 200 mg a day. Increase the dose slowly only if safe to do so.

L Phenylalanine is best taken on an empty stomach with water or juice about an hour before meals. High-protein foods, in particular, can interfere with proper absorption.

Handy Tip

At recommended doses, DLPA occasionally causes mild side effects, such as heartburn, nausea, or headaches. This can be prevented by taking it with a glass of water. At excessive doses (more than 1.5g a day), it can cause numbness, tingling, or other signs of nerve damage over a period of time

L Proline

Tips for absorption

Synergistic nutrients are magnesium, B6 and niacin

Taurine

Tips for absorption

Taurine is found in pre and post workout formulas, and in sugar laden energy drinks, so the general consensus is out on the best time to take it and whether it needs an insulin spike or not to allow it to enter cells.

L Threonine

Tips for absorption

Synergistic nutrients are magnesium, B6 and niacin.

L Tryptophan

For anxiety, depression and sleep, take 1hr-30 mins before bed.

Tips for solubility

Low degree heated water (up to 30 degrees) will aid solubility. Excessive heating is not recommended as it will affect the stability of the product.

Tyrosine

Tips for neurotransmitter production

L-Tyrosine should be taken before meals, preferably 30 minutes before, and divided into two or three doses daily.

Tyrosine supplements are best taken with a B group or multivitamin/mineral complex because vitamins B6, B9, folic acid and the copper mineral help in the conversion of L-Tyrosine into neurotransmitters

Hygroscopic Amino Acids

Some amino acids when combined with others either smell offensively or attract water rendering the entire complex unstable.

Smelly and hygroscopic amino acids are Cysteine, N-Acetyl Cysteine, choline and to a lesser extent Methionine.

These amino acids may be compounded with other if a dehydrating agent is added like silica. I prefer to compound these amino acids separately and not adulterate the compound with unnecessary additives.

Amino Acid Base formula

Amino acids custom compounded blend contains a base formula to supply all essential amino acids required for optimal physiological function.

The base formula constitutes a certain percentage of the blend with the bulk remainder making up amino acids that are deficient in lab results.

Catabolism of body protein may contribute relatively small amounts of essential amino acids to blood and urine.

Estimated daily essential amino acid requirements

Amino Acid	Adults (mg/kg body weight)	Estimated for a 60kg adult (mg)	Amount (mg) provided by 44g serve
Histidine	10	600	663
Isoleucine	20	1200	1247
Leucine	39	2340	2572
Lysine	30	1800	884
Methionine	10	600	868
Phenylalanine + Tyrosine	25	1500	3147 (1604 + 1543)
Threonine	15	900	1062
Tryptophan	4	240	387
Valine	26	1560	1846

Adapted from Table 23: Summary of the adult indispensable amino acid requirements. In: Joint WHO/FAO/UNU Expert Consultation. Protein and amino acid requirements in human nutrition (WHO technical report series; no.935, p.510). Geneva: WHO, 2007.

Dr Erdman has formulated a base formula based of the magnificent egg. This base formula is best suited to an amino acid supplement with consideration for all deficient amino acids.

Note that cofactors are needed for amino acid metabolism. Take special note of the co-factors when amino acid results are elevated.

Power of Amino Acids in the Magnificent Egg

The egg contains higher lecithin content and other nutrients which does not raise blood cholesterol levels contrary to previous reports. To consider cholesterol content only is misleading because the ratio of cholesterol to other nutrients is important.

Recent studies have shown that high intake of sugar and junk foods raises blood sugar and cholesterol levels despite its low cholesterol content.

Most foods contain a few essential amino acids which are called limiting amino acids for that food. The protein will be utilized by the body only to the extent that the limiting amino acid is present. The egg wonderful balance of amino acids makes its proteins more usable than most other sources.

Egg consumption fluctuates due the suspected contribution to heart attacks. The maligned egg is possibly the perfect amino acid source.

The base amino acid formula is formulated in accordance with the protein content of the humble egg.

Steak or red meats are often considered great sources of amino acids which tends to raise amino acids Lysine, Valine, Threonine and Leucine to very high levels.

Amino acid base formulas derived from the amino acid content of an egg and suggests ways to achieve a more balanced amino acid level. At present the egg is probably the best amino acid food source.

Cautions and Precautions

Amino acids are found in the diet and taken daily in the diet. However, some amino acids may need to be used with caution.

Tyrosine and Phenylalanine can inhibit one another's passage into the brain.

Taurine and Glycine have the same function and compete for absorption.

Glutamic acid and Aspartic acid have the same function and compete for absorption, but have a function opposite to that of Taurine and Glycine. Thus glutamic acid can promote absorption of Glycine and Taurine, and Glycine can promote absorption of glutamic acid.

Some amino acids interact with drug. Tyrosine metabolism is inhibited by tranquilizer, haloperidol and hypertensive, methyl L-dopa.

Concurrent use of Arginine with antihypertensive medication may potentiate hypotensive effects.

Glycine may exacerbate symptoms when taken with clozapine or other atypical antipsychotics.

Use of selective serotonin reuptake inhibitors (SSRIs), tricyclic antidepressants or monoamine oxidase inhibitors (MAOIs) with Tryptophan may increase the risk of serotonergic side effects.

Tyramine-containing foods should be avoided while on MAOIs.

Inborn Errors of Metabolism

More than 70 inherited amino acidopathies are now known, all falling into two general classes:
- enzymatic defects in amino acid catabolism
- disorders of transmembrane transport.

The catabolic defects far outnumber the transport abnormalities.

Most of these disorders are rare, their incidences ranging from 1 in 12,000 for Phenylketonuria (PKU) although rare in incidence is associated with Phenylalanine metabolism abnormalities. Most common is homocystinuria associated with amino acids metabolism, namely Methionine abnormalities.[59]

Symptoms range from none to severe neurological dysfunction, and they are usually prevented or mitigated by appropriate dietary amino acid restriction or vitamin supplementation.

Mild cystinuria, a renal transport disorder, has been observed in allergy and may occur in the general population with an incidence of 1 in 400. This condition is usually accompanied by renal excretion of Lysine, Ornithine and Arginine.[60]

In Conclusion

The study of amino acids is vast and, at the same time simplistic. I do hope that you use **"Alchemy of Amino acids" e-book** in line with **"Alchemy amino acids Masterclass"** to enhance the health of your patients.

I am most grateful to my esteemed peer's Dr Richard Lord, Dr Alexandra Bralley, and Dr Eric Braverman for their insightful research and availability of their texts. As the purpose of this book and masterclass is to provide a simplistic practical application of amino acids in your clinical practice, detailed biochemistry has been omitted.

Please consult with texts listed in the reference for further information.

Amino Acids are powerful healers, use them!

Acknowledgments

I would like to thank my peers for their former dedication and work on Amino Acids in texts they have researched and written.

In particular, I wish to thank my gurus in Amino Acids!

Dr Richard S Lord and Dr J. Alexandra Bralley in their text "Laboratory evaluations for Integrative and functional Medicine". This text is well researched and jam packed with detailed biochemistry with an in-depth understanding of integrative medicine.

"The Amino Revolution" by Robert Erdmann. Dr Erdmann's work was the trigger for my interest in Amino Acids. His simplistic view and practical use of amino acids for therapeutic use sparked my interest to learn more.

"The healing nutrients within" by Dr Eric R Braverman

"Amino Acid Compendium" by Ilve Hunt. Ilve has kindly provided with permission from KRPAN enterprises to include Amino Acids compendium in this text.

References

With much gratitude from my esteemed peers!

The texts I have used in the compilation of this text are:

Dr R. Lord and Dr J A. Bralley – *Laboratory evaluations in Integrative medicine*

Dr Eric Braverman - *Healing nutrients within*

Dr Erdman – *The Amino Revolution*

Ilve Hunt - *The Amino Acid Compendium*

www.aminoacidsguide.com

www.examine.com

1. Francesco S. Dioguardi, Clinical use of amino acids as dietary supplement: pros and cons, J Cachexia Sarcopenia Muscle. 2011 Jun; 2(2): 75–80.
2. Adapted from "The healing nutrients within" by Dr Eric Braverman
3. Chromiak JA1, Antonio J. Use of amino acids as growth hormone-releasing agents by athletes. Nutrition. 2002 Jul-Aug;18(7-8):657-61.
4. Fairhall KM1et al, Central effects of growth hormone-releasing hexapeptide (GHRP-6) on growth hormone release are inhibited by central somatostatin action. J Endocrinol. 1995 Mar;144(3):555-60.
5. Borsheim et al, Am J Physiol Endocrin Metab Oct 2002; 383(4)E468-657

6. Waziri R, Wilcox J, Sherman AD, Mott J. Serine metabolism and psychosis. Psychiatry Res. 1984 Jun;12(2):121-36.

7. Shigeri Y1, Shimamoto K. Nihon Yakurigaku Zasshi. Pharmacology of excitatory amino acid transporters (EAATs and VGLUTs) 2003 Sep;122(3):253-64.

8. Dong-Hee Kim,1et al, Effect of BCAA intake during endurance exercises on fatigue substances, muscle damage substances, and energy metabolism substances, J Exerc Nutrition Biochem. 2013 Dec; 17(4): 169–180.

9. J H Koeslag, T D Noakes, and A W Sloan, The effects of Alanine, glucose and starch ingestion on the ketosis produced by exercise and by starvation. J Physiol. 1982; 325: 363–376.

10. R. M. Hobson et al, Effects of β-Alanine supplementation on exercise performance: a meta-analysis, Amino Acids. 2012 Jul; 43(1): 25–37.

11. B.I. Campbell, P.M. La Bounty, M. Roberts. The Ergogenic Potential of Arginine. J Int Soc Sports Nutr, 1 (2) (2004), pp. 35-38.

12. Naseh Pahlavan et al, L-Arginine supplementation and risk factors of cardiovascular diseases in healthy men, PMID: 28751963

13. Willoughby DS et al, Effects of 7 days of Arginine-alpha-ketoglutarate supplementation on blood flow, plasma L-Arginine, nitric oxide metabolites, and asymmetric dimethyl Arginine after resistance exercise. Int J Sport Nutr Exerc Metab. 2011 Aug;21(4):291-9.

14. Mukundh N. Balasubramanian et al, Asparagine synthetase: regulation by cell stress and involvement in tumor biology, Am J Physiol Endocrinol Metab. 2013 Apr 15; 304(8): E789–E799.

15. Geoffrey W Melville et al, Three and six g supplementation of d-Aspartic acid in resistance trained men, J Int Soc Sports Nutr. 2015; 12: 15.

16. Brandsch C1, Eder K. Effect of L-carnitine on weight loss and body composition of rats fed a hypocaloric diet. Ann Nutr Metab. 2002;46(5):205-10.

17. Spagnoli A et al, Long-term acetyl-L-carnitine treatment in Alzheimer's disease. Neurology. 1991 Nov;41(11):1726-32.

18. Steven H. Zeisel, Choline: An Essential Nutrient for Public Health, Nutr Rev. 2009 Nov; 67(11): 615–623.

References

19. Bendahan D1 et al, Citrulline/malate promotes aerobic energy production in human exercising muscle. Br J Sports Med. 2002 Aug;36(4):282-9.

20. Kreider RB1 Effects of Creatine supplementation on performance and training adaptations. Mol Cell Biochem. 2003 Feb;244(1-2):89-94.

21. Schmaal L, Efficacy of N-acetylCysteine in the treatment of nicotine dependence: a double-blind placebo-controlled pilot study. Eur Addict Res. 2011;17(4):211-6.

22. Vida Mokhtari, A Review on Various Uses of N-Acetyl Cysteine ,Cell J. 2017 Apr-Jun; 19(1): 11–17.

23. Grigorian et al, N-Acetylglucosamine Inhibits T-helper 1 (Th1)/T-helper 17 (Th17) Cell Responses Ani, J Biol Chem. 2011 Nov 18; 286(46): 40133–40141.

24. Lydiard RB1. The role of GABA in anxiety disorders. J Clin Psychiatry. 2003;64 Suppl 3:21-7.

25. Min-Hyun Kim et al, The Roles of Glutamine in the Intestine and Its Implication in Intestinal Diseases, Int J Mol Sci. 2017 May; 18(5): 1051.

26. Gannon MC et al, The metabolic response to ingested Glycine. Am J Clin Nutr. 2002 Dec;76(6):1302-7.

27. Vittorio Unfer et al, Myo-Inositol effects in women with PCOS: a meta-analysis of randomized controlled trials, Endocr Connect. 2017 Nov; 6(8): 647–658.

28. Westhof E, Flossmann W, Müller A. The action of ionizing radiation on protein: radical formation in L-Histidine crystals. Int J Radiat Biol Relat Stud Phys Chem Med. 1975 Jan;27(1):51-62.

29. L Breen and T A Churchward-Venne, Leucine: a nutrient 'trigger' for muscle anabolism, but what more? J Physiol. 2012 May; 590(Pt 9): 2065–2066.

30. Griffith RS et al, Success of L-Lysine therapy in frequently recurrent herpes simplex infection. Treatment and prophylaxis. Dermatologica. 1987;175(4):183-90.

31. Kim SH et al, Comparative study of fatty liver induced by Methionine and choline-deficiency in C57BL/6N mice originating from three different sources. Lab Anim Res. 2017 Jun;33(2):157-164. doi: 10.5625/lar.2017.33.2.157. Epub 2017 Jun 30.

32. Zajac A et al, Arginine and Ornithine supplementation increases growth hormone and insulin-like growth factor-1 serum levels after heavy-resistance exercise in strength-trained athletes. J Strength Cond Res. 2010 Apr;24(4):1082-90.

33. Walsh NE et al, Analgesic effectiveness of D-Phenylalanine in chronic pain patients. Arch Phys Med Rehabil. 1986 Jul;67(7):436-9.

34. Barbul A, Proline precursors to sustain Mammalian collagen synthesis. J Nutr. 2008 Oct;138(10):2021S-2024S.

35. Yukihiko Ito et al, Effects of L-Serine ingestion on human sleep Springerplus. 2014; 3: 456. 2014 Aug 22. doi: 10.1186/2193-1801-3-456

36. Biemans EA, Verhoeven-Duif NM, Gerrits J et al. (2016) CSF d-Serine concentrations are similar in Alzheimer's disease, other dementias, and elderly controls. Neurobiol Aging 42, 213-216.

37. Weng J et al, Diabetes Metabolism: Research and Reviews--Chinese Diabetes Society special issue: a small but encouraging step toward the successful control of diabetes in China. Diabetes Metab Res Rev. 2014 Sep;30(6):445-6

38. Yan-Jun Xu et al, The potential health benefits of Taurine in cardiovascular disease, Exp Clin Cardiol. 2008 Summer; 13(2): 57–65.

39. Wu GF et al, Antidepressant effect of Taurine in chronic unpredictable mild stress-induced depressive rats. Sci Rep. 2017 Jul 10;7(1):4989

40. Nobre AC et al, L-Theanine, a natural constituent in tea, and its effect on mental state. Asia Pac J Clin Nutr. 2008;17 Suppl 1:167-8.

41. Stephen L. Hauser et al, Arch Neurol. An Antispasticity Effect of Threonine in Multiple Sclerosis 1992;49(9):923-926

42. Schneider-Helmert D, Spinweber CL. Evaluation of L-Tryptophan for treatment of insomnia: a review. Psychopharmacology (Berl). 1986;89(1):1-7.

43. Simon N. Young, L-Tyrosine to alleviate the effects of stress? J Psychiatry Neurosci. 2007 May; 32(3): 224.

44. Fasching P, et al. Insulin production following intravenous glucose, Arginine, and Valine: different pattern in patients with impaired glucose tolerance and non-insulin-dependent diabetes mellitus. Metabolism. (1994)

References

45. al-Damluji S et al, Adrenergic control of the secretion of anterior pituitary hormones. Baillieres Clin Endocrinol Metab. 1993 Apr;7(2):355-92.

46. Bell KM, Potkin SG, Carreon D, Plon L. S-adenosylMethionine blood levels in major depression: changes with drug treatment. Acta Neurol Scand Suppl 1994;154:15-18.

47. Reinstein DK, Lehnert H, Wurtman RJ. Dietary Tyrosine suppresses the rise in plasma corticosterone following acute stress in rats. Life Sci 1985;37(23):2157-2163.

48. Fendt SM et al, Neurons eat Glutamate to stay alive. J Cell Biol. 2017 Apr 3;216(4):863-865.

49. Torok, O., and Csaba, G., Effect of glutaTaurine, a newly discovered parathyroid hormone on rat thymus cultures. Acta Morphol. Acad. Sci. Hung., 26(2):87-94, 1978.

50. Fisman M, Gordon B, Feleki V, Helmes E, Appell J, Rabheru K. Hyperammonemia in Alzheimer's disease. Am J Psychiatry 1985; 142(1):71-73.

51. Scriver CR, Gibson K. Disorders of Beta and Gamma Amino Acids in Free and Peptide-linked Forms. In: Scriver C, Beaudet A, Sly W, Valle D, editors. The metabolic and molecular bases of inherited disease. Vol 1. 7th Ed. New York: McGraw-Hill Book Company, 1995: 1349- 1370. Crabbe P, Isselbacher KJ. Urinary hydroxyProline excretion in malabsorption states:. Gastroenterology 1965;48(3):307-311.

52. María M. Adeva-Andany et al, Liver glucose metabolism in humans, Biosci Rep. 2016 Dec; 36(6).

53. Timbrell JA. Toxic responses to foreign compounds. In: Principles of biochemical toxicology, 2nd ed. London and Bristol, PA: Taylor & Francis Inc, 1994:221-232.

54. Guoyao Wu et al, Proline and hydroxyProline metabolism: implications for animal and human nutrition, Amino Acids. 2011 Apr; 40(4): 1053–1063.

55. Kinscherf R, Fischbach T, Mihm S, Roth S, Hohenhaus-Sievert E, Weiss C, et al. Effect of glutathione depletion and oral N-acetyl Cysteine treatment on CD4+ and CD8+ cells. FASEB J 1994;8(6):448-451. 30 Jeevanandam M, Young DH, Ramias L, Schiller WR. Amino aciduria of severe trauma. Am J Clin Nutr 1989;49:815-822.

56. Brattstrom L, Lindgren A, Israelsson B, Malinow MR, Norrving B, Upson B, et al. Hyperhomocysteinaemia in stroke: prevalence, cause, and relationships to type of stroke and stroke risk factors. Eur J Clin Invest 1992; 22(3):214-221.

57. Ulrich Förstermann et al, Nitric oxide synthases: regulation and function, Eur Heart J. 2012 Apr; 33(7): 829–837.

58. Lab evaluations for integrative and functional medicine by J Bralley and R Lord

59. Pangborn J. Amino acid analysis and therapy: opportunities and pitfills. Vol 1. 7th ed. New York: McGraw-Hill, Inc, 1995:5-9.

60. Hank J, Treatment options in energetic, functional, biologic medicine. Syllabus for the Great Lakes College of Clinical Medicine Symposium; 1997 Feb 28-Mar 2; Asheville (NC):7.